# *Dieting Makes You Fat*

# Dieting Makes You Fat

## A guide to energy, fitness and health

*Geoffrey Cannon and Hetty Einzig*

C

CENTURY PUBLISHING
LONDON

First published in Great Britain in 1983
by Century Publishing Co. Ltd,
76 Old Compton Street, London W1V 5PA

ISBN 0 7126 0118 X

Reproduced, printed and bound in Great Britain by
Hazell Watson & Viney Ltd, Aylesbury, Bucks

*ετον ετελιο καλαμαρα*
*και καλαμαρακια*

# *Preface*

This is not a diet book. It is a book about dieting. It is also a guide to human energy, fitness and health.

By 'diet' and 'dieting' we are not referring to the quality of what people eat, because of their habits, beliefs or desire for health (as in 'vegetarian diet'). We are referring to the quantity, or rather lack of quantity, of food eaten, because of a desire to lose weight (as in 'calorie-controlled diet'). When we say that dieting makes you fat, we are using the word 'diet' in the sense of diet regime.

This book is not for people who are very fat indeed, who may, unfortunately, be suffering from a metabolic disorder and need special hospital treatment. A woman of normal height weighing, say, 18 stone, or more, may need to be starved and kept under medical supervision in order to regain health. We are writing for people who are not ill; for the scores of millions of people in the West who are fatter than they want to be, who have tried dieting, who have found that dieting does not work, and who want to know why.

We do not recommend the use of drugs as a means to lose weight. It is our conviction, shared by doctors who have supported us in the preparation of this book, that now is the time for people in the West to take responsibility for their own health and to avoid drugs whenever possible. Able-bodied people do not need drugs to lose weight, and any drug devised to suppress appetite or to speed up metabolism is liable to be as damaging to health as is nicotine and the other poisons in cigarettes.

The research for this book has been the joint responsibility of the two authors. The book has been written by Geoffrey Cannon, and the 'I' throughout the book is therefore his; with the exception of chapters 6 and 7, which are written from a woman's view by Hetty Einzig.

# Acknowledgements

Sir Douglas Black, Dr Denis Craddock, Professor John Durnin, Dr Katherine Elliott, Dr Elizabeth Ferris, Dr Kenneth Heaton and Professor Peter Wood read the book, or pertinent sections of it, and gave us encouragement and advice which we have incorporated for publication.

Professor Per-Olof Åstrand, Dr David Booth, Dr Denis Burkitt, Ben Cannon, Dr Kenneth Cooper, Susan Einzig, Malcolm Emery, Dr John Garrow, Dr Oliver Gillie, Victoria Huxley, Professor Harry Keen, Dr Derrick Lonsdale, Mary Mackintosh, Tom McNab, Dr Alan Maryon Davis, David Nabarro, Alison Paul, Dr David Player, Dr David Ryde, Aubrey Sheiham, Professor Albert Stunkard, Dr Hugh Trowell, Professor Arvid Wretlind, Professor John Yudkin and Dr John Yudkin gave us advice or guidance on particular aspects of the book.

We owe special thanks to everyone who helped us. The responsibility for views expressed in the book is of course ours. We will be glad to hear from any reader who wishes to contradict or to amplify any points we make.

The climate that has made it possible for us to prepare the book has been created by friends, colleagues, and by workers in the field, whom we would also like to acknowledge.

At the *Sunday Times*, John Lovesey and Norman Harris have championed the cause of fitness and health for all. At *Running* magazine, Sylvester Stein, Alison Turnbull, and especially Andy Etchells, have supported the projects that turned some of the thinking behind the book into living experience. Cardiologists Dr Robin Hedworth-Whitty and Dr Peter Williams, together with physiologists Ted Charlesworth and Kevin Sykes, and Dick Hubbard, Rita Rowe and Ian Jamieson, supported these projects. At the Bodyworkshop Barbara Dale, Catherine Mackwood and Esme Newton-Dunn have shared their experience and enthusiasm.

For the *London 1982/50* project, special thanks are due to Will Chapman, Jim Cockburn, Rosemary Evison, John Goody, Joyce Goody, Michael Jacob, Hilda Nyman, Rosemary Tempest, and John Walker; to Terry Bennett, Peter Bird, Don Clark, Steven Downes, James Kelly, Ken Walker and Stan Weber; and above all to Simon Morris. For the *Fun Runner '82* project, as well as those already mentioned, special thanks are due to Bill Brown, James Godber, Dr Barrie Gunter, Mick Rankin, Bernie Tuck and Wendy Wood; and to Allan Appleton, Vic Burrowes, Tim Burton, Vivienne Coady, Bill East, Jane Heywood, Michael Innes, Rodney Lewis, Teresa Malinowska, Liz Parry, Bobbie Randall, John Routledge and Eileen Ward. For the *Getting in Shape* project, special thanks are due to Professor David Denison, Malcolm Emery, Dr Bob Green, Jane Howarth, Tom McNab, Dr Andy Peacock, Bev Risman, and the staff at the National Heart and Chest Hospital and the West London Institute; and above all to Will Chapman. Everyone connected with these projects is to be thanked; some three times over.

Personal support was given by Kathy Crilley, Corinne McLuhan, Teri McLuhan, Charlotte Parry-Crooke, Rosalind Schwartz, and by our families.

Sir Douglas Black, President of the Royal College of Physicians of London, will be remembered for three reports, on Medical Aspects of Dietary Fibre, Inequalities in Health, and Obesity, all of which have influenced us. Inspiration and encouragement has also been given by Graham Alexander, Dr June Burger, Helen Davis, Bob Donovan, John Falkiner, Tim Gallwey, John Gravelle, Bob Kriegel, Ian McGarry, Michael Murphy, John Poppy, John Ridgway, Mark Shapiro, Paul Spangler, Leslie Watson and Sir John Whitmore, all of whom have contributed some spirit to the book.

Professor Marshall McLuhan became a dear friend and a teacher who encouraged the knowledge that progress often requires looking a paradox in the eye. The book is the poorer for having been written after his death.

Deborah Rogers, our agent, and Gail Rebuck, our publisher, together with Anthony Cheetham, had the courage of our conviction. We owe special thanks to them.

# *Contents*

# Introduction

In January 1983 the Royal College of Physicians of London published a report on obesity. Commenting on surveys of British men and women in the last 50 years the report states: 'There now seems little doubt that there is a general trend for both men and women to become heavier and presumably fatter, this change being particularly evident in young adults.

In common with the citizens of the USA and other Western countries, British people are getting fatter. According to the 1981 Census, about a quarter of men and women in their 20s and just under half the population over 40 are carrying excess weight. If you assume that these figures merely demonstrate that we are eating more, they will not surprise you. But we are eating less. British government statistics show that since 1960 we have consumed a steadily decreasing amount of energy from food and drink.

It is generally assumed that fat people are greedy and, certainly, that they not only eat too much but also more than lean people. How could it be otherwise? In 1982 Alison Paul, a leading nutritionist, reported that British children and teenagers are eating less than their parents, are consuming anything from 300 to 500 calories a day less than World Health Organisation recommendations, yet are more likely to be overweight than underweight. Professor Harry Keen of Guy's Hospital conducted a survey of 3,000 adults which showed that those who ate most had least body fat. And in 1983 Professor Peter Wood of

Stanford University in California, reporting on studies carried out in Britain, the USA and other Western countries, said 'Generally speaking, fatter people eat less than thinner people.'

### Diets slow you down

These facts are not well known simply because they are so puzzling. I have yet to read them in any diet book. This is no surprise, because they suggest what millions of dieters have found out for themselves: that diets do not work.

An older generation used to say that fat people were unlucky, because they had 'something wrong with their glands'. A more sophisticated version used the word 'genes' rather than 'glands'. A theory which went the rounds recently is that fat people are stuck with a 'set-point' programmed to make them fat. This is a variation of an older idea, that fat people are lumbered with a 'low metabolism'. From the point of view of the fat person who wants to be thin, all these theories are bad news. They all imply that there is not much anyone can do about being fat; that some people are born to be thin, others born to be fat, and, well, there it is.

But these notions cannot be right for one reason alone: the example of non-Western societies. People living in settled rural communities untouched by Western influence often live to a ripe old age and eat well without becoming overweight, let alone obese. Moreover, before the Industrial Revolution few people other than the rich in Western countries became fat. The theory that, all of a sudden, fatness became inherited is absurd.

Every book on dieting tells you to concentrate on reducing the amount of energy you take in from food. And most will tell you that, while exercise is good for you, it won't make much difference to your weight. Stay sedentary but go on a diet, is the message. But recent studies have shown that active people are leaner and lighter than sedentary people, and lose weight as a result of exercise. And, also, active people eat much more food than sedentary people.

When we talk of 'metabolism' or, more correctly, 'metabolic rate' we are referring to the speed at which the body uses energy. The diet books assume that while different people have different metabolic rates, every individual has a fixed rate. That is to say, we are taught that we are stuck with the metabolic rate we are born with. And dieters are also led to believe that most if not all weight lost on a diet, is fat. But scientists have known for more than 50 years that dieting slows the body down and certain types of exercise speed it up: well established facts that, if published in diet books, would damage their sales.

This was the point at which Hetty Einzig and I began the research for this book. And we came to realise that, much more often than not, dieting creates the conditions it is meant to cure. That is to say, dieting makes you fat.

Some diet books claim that their regimes can make you lose 10 pounds or more in a week. This claim is accurate. But the weight lost is not fat. It is glycogen, a form of glucose bound up with water, stored in the muscles and liver, which is the immediately available energy needed by the body and brain. Loss of glycogen triggers intense sensations of hunger. Once a diet regime is ended the glycogen will be replaced. Have you ever read that in a diet book?

## Exercise speeds you up

The exciting news is that metabolic rate is not static: it is dynamic. Within wide limits we can choose the speed at which we want our bodies to work, and we can gain a faster metabolic rate by the right kind of exercise. The body gradually adapts to endurance exercise by losing fat and gaining lean tissue. This training effect allows us to eat more while losing fat because working muscle is very much more metabolically active than body fat.

It is only in the past few years, as a result of the running and aerobics boom in the USA, Great Britain and other Western countries, that millions of people have changed from being overweight dieters, to leaner, lighter, fit and healthy people, who exercise a lot and eat a lot too.

Diet books tell us to worry about the quantity of the food we eat, on the assumption that the basic requirement of the body is energy from food. This assumption is wrong too. The basic requirement of the body is not for quantity but for quality. What is wrong with the food we eat is its lack of quality; what the body needs is not so much energy as nourishment.

### Good food—the recipe for health

More and more doctors are now acknowledging that the diseases of the gut that so many of us suffer and die from are often caused by eating processed foods, the chief of which is refined sugar; and that heart disease and other ailments are often caused by inactivity. The sedentary dieter, who eats least food of all, leads an unhealthy life. The sedentary person who does eat enough nourishing food is liable to gain fat, simply because the only way to get enough nourishment from food is to consume too much energy.

The solution is that you can lose fat and also help yourself to good health by eating well and leading an active life: a remedy that many family doctors once recommended, but which has now been largely forgotten. It is our conviction that dieting is not only self-defeating but also a means whereby tens of millions of men, and at least twice as many women, are prevented from enjoying their own lives.

You can change your life only when you know that you are able to make the change. Dieters often feel helpless not only about their weight and shape but about their lives; because they do not know how to become the shape and weight that is right for them. This book may encourage you to take your life back into your own hands.

# CHAPTER ONE

# Confessions of a Dieter

A man or woman may live and work and maintain bodily equilibrium on either a higher or lower energy level. One essential question is, what level is most advantageous? The answer to this must be sought not only in metabolism experiments and dietary studies, but also in broader observations regarding bodily and mental efficiency and general health, strength and welfare.

W O ATWATER AND F G BENEDICT
*Bulletin of the US Department of Agriculture*, 1902


Quality. You know what it is, yet you don't know what it is. But that's self-contradictory. But some things *are* better than others, that is, they have more quality. But when you try to say what the quality is, apart from the things that have it, it all goes poof! . . . Obviously some things are better than others, but what's the *betterness*?

ROBERT C PIRSIG
*Zen and the Art of Motorcycle Maintenance*


## Memoirs of a failed dieter

I found a slip of paper recently, folded into an old wallet. It read:

**2 eggs boiled or poached**
**4 ounces of lean meat OR boiled fish**
**1 slice bread**
**2 water biscuits**
**½ ounce butter (level dessert spoon)**

½ ounce sugar (level dessert spoon)
1 ounce milk (two coffees white)
2 ounces hard cheese

in any amount:
water (three pints at least)
tea, coffee
gherkins, dry spices
peppers (only 'fruit' allowed)
lemon
chemical sweeteners
green salad (only vegetables allowed)

all else forbidden, including:
butter + ½ ounce
sugar + ½ ounce
alcohol
fruit, fruit juice

Dieting connoisseurs will recognise this daily regime as a version of the high-protein diets set out in *The Doctor's Quick Weight Loss Diet* by Dr Irwin Stillman and in *The Complete Scarsdale Medical Diet* by the late Dr Herman Tarnower. My version was sterner about fruit and vegetables, and cheated a bit with the butter and sugar.

Dr Stillman and Dr Tarnower disagree in some respects. But a lot of people believe in their diet regimes; to date, their books have sold a total of twenty million copies, worldwide. 'I'm convinced that the Quick Weight Loss Diet is the finest and best for most people who should take off excess weight,' wrote Dr Stillman in 1967. 'No diet has ever been as spontaneously and unanimously acclaimed as this one,' wrote Dr Tarnower in 1978. He went further: 'I urge you to get started now on this diet. Every day that you delay and keep or increase that extra poundage is impairing your appearance and your health, and is endangering and shortening your life. Overweight is a kind of death for almost everyone, slow for some, quicker for others.' Fervent words.

## Weight lost—and regained

I first tried the high-protein diet in 1970. It worked. My weight came down from 13 stone 8 pounds to 10 stone 9 in twelve weeks. I had reached and passed my target.

In 1974 I went on the high-protein diet again. This time I followed the word of Stillman more faithfully, adding fruit, vegetables, tuna with all the oil drained, diet soda, and mustard to the regime. I cut out sugar and butter but allowed myself one sin—a glass of wine. It worked again. This time my weight came down from 12 stone 12 pounds to 12 stone 2 in two weeks; to 11 stone 6 pounds in four weeks; then the rate of loss slowed so that after six weeks I was 11 stone 1. Then, after nine weeks, by a dizzying and ecstatic effort of will I broke the 150-pound barrier; and held steady at 10 stone 6 between weeks twelve and sixteen.

Like psychiatrists and schoolteachers, diet doctors often have a way of suggesting that if all goes according to plan the credit is theirs, whereas if you fail the fault is yours. I believed them. I had regained 2 stone 3 pounds between 1970 and 1974, despite two intermediate purges each of 12 pounds. And, by New Year's Day 1976, I had regained 2 stone 4 pounds. At midnight I made a New Year resolution and, for a week, followed the regime set down in Dr Allan Cott's *The Ultimate Diet* and in Shirley Ross's *The Super Diet*. I fasted. Not a pea. Just water. Well, a small sin: milk in coffee.

After three days, I found, as the books said, that hunger faded, and I felt clean, light-headed and sharpened. More to the point, after ten days I had lost 15 pounds, finishing up at 11 stone 9. But, by the end of April, I had regained 16 pounds.

My biggest weight loss was on a 'single-food' diet. These diets, often touted as fun, do not count calories but restrict the dieter to one (or a few) foods. The more ingenious versions stipulate a food normally seen as a treat, which, in due course, you come to hate. Examples are the grapefruit diet, the milk and banana diet and the ice-cream diet. Single-food diets are usually sold along with some mumbo-jumbo about the special qualities of the food to be eaten.

Judy Mazel's 'Beverly Hills Diet' is a skilfully marketed version of the single-food diet. It restricts the dieter to exotic fruits (mango, papaya, with pineapple) for days at a time. Since the average-sized woman would have to eat 8 pounds of mangoes a day to supply her normal energy requirement, it is hardly surprising that the Beverly Hills Diet works.

### Ten-potato diet

Any single-food diet will work, whatever the food. In a classic experiment—of rather more nutritional significance than Ms Mazel's diet—twenty-three young Irishmen from Galway, organised by Dr Denis Burkitt, volunteered to eat ten large potatoes baked in their skins every day for three months. Most of them lost weight, for the potatoes represented about 1000 calories a day, much less energy than the body normally needs for its maintenance. No one yet has become rich and famous propagating this Irish diet, which is surprising in a way, since the volunteers were told that they could eat anything they liked every day, after they had eaten the potatoes. In the event they found they had little room left for pork chops or profiteroles.

My own version of the single-food diet was oranges—with the occasional tomato. The principle of this regime was that I liked oranges and tomatoes; and still do, surprisingly enough. In three months in 1967 I dropped almost 3 stone, from 13 stone 3 pounds to 10 stone 4. I celebrated by buying a suit, which fitted me for two days and which still hangs in my wardrobe, a memento of two days in my life when I was thin.

I was good at dieting. I could always win a lose-weight contest. My first epic diet was of the 'sensible' type recommended by Professor John Yudkin in his book *This Slimming Business* and, more recently, by the Consumers' Association in *Which? Way to Slim*: low carbohydrates; cut down, or out, bread, pasta, cereals, confectionery, cakes, biscuits, potatoes and alcohol. 'A low-carbohydrate diet is good for general health, not only for slimming,' says the *Which?* guide. This worked too: I lost 1 stone

10 pounds, which I regained in two years. It was, as I recall, this failure that led me to try most other diets, once. Nevertheless, on two or three other occasions I cut out the carbohydrates, regarding bread and potatoes, with sweets, as bad, and would lose 7 to 10 pounds in two or three weeks.

Between 1964 and 1976 I lost about 200 pounds. If all my diets had worked, on New Year's Day 1976 I would have weighed minus 20 pounds. But the records I kept were full of notes like 'half-way there!' and then 'failed' and 'failed again'. Most of my life consisted of backsliding from diets. Was it the spoon of sugar, the glass of wine? I supposed that between diet regimes I 'let go'; I felt bound to agree with Professor Yudkin:

> The upshot is that if you take too much food, containing too much fat and carbohydrate (or to a much lesser extent too much protein) you will be piling up an excess which you will store as fat . . . . In the end, it is food, and only food, that makes you overweight.

I read this as meaning that I was greedy. Gaining weight was a visible sign of an inward weakness; of a general failure as a person. If I didn't diet I feared and believed that I would balloon up and become like the Michelin Man. These horrid fantasies drove me to diet regimes. Dieting is a private matter. Like 'dirty' books, diet books are not read in public places, because in both cases people are ashamed to reveal how they fall short of what is expected of them and what they want to expect of themselves. The best-selling British paperback of 1982 was Audrey Eyton's *The F-Plan Diet*, recommending fibre as a means to slim, which to date has sold 1,600,000 copies and has sold faster than any other British paperback except *Lady Chatterley's Lover*. But when I was a dieter in the 1970s I thought I was alone with my problems.


### *Trying psychology*

I tried psychology. On another slip of paper I wrote 'Being Fat Means'

Clothes don't fit. Good clothes hang, wasted, in the wardrobe. I pretend drab and baggy clothes are best.

I get tired, especially at weekends. I loll around listlessly, and may even sleep in the afternoons.

Food is obsessive. I eat, feel bloated, and then feel hungry again. I look for eating companions.

Embarrassment. In clothes shops, on a beach, with friends, playing cricket, seeing people after a gap.

Depression. At lack of self-control, at evidence of middle age, at knowledge of impaired health.

Gaining weight and being fat appeared to be my most intractable personal problem. I hated myself physically and despised my ineffectiveness. I didn't shape up. When I crossed the 180-pound line, self-respect or self-hatred would motivate me, and I'd go on another diet regime. Dieting was my dirty little secret. But my greed was a vice I couldn't keep to myself. It showed.

In 1978 the consumer magazine *Which?* surveyed 1001 slimmers, 788 women and 213 men. The main single reason given for failure as a dieter was 'lack of willpower and determination'. 'I know how to lose weight. I know I can lose weight. I lack the willpower to keep at it for what amounts to a lifetime, because whenever I give up on the programme I put it on again,' said one respondent. And another, 'I am very good at losing weight but once the loss slows down I give up and tend to put it all back on again.' As for me, two couplets by Theodore Roethke came to mind:

Self-contemplation is a curse
That makes an old confusion worse.
He who himself begins to loathe
Grows sick in flesh and spirit both.

But what to do? I ate, I wanted food, I grew fat. Food, hunger, appetite, my body, were my enemies.

## *Too much energy in, too little out*

Diet books usually say that fat people either eat too much or take too little exercise. That seems common sense enough. So, I thought, maybe my vice was not greed, but sloth. Most diet books do not, however, forecast a slim future for the fat exerciser. 'It is extremely difficult to lose significant weight by exercise,' says Dr Tarnower. 'A half hour of energetic bicycling, for instance, uses up 200-280 calories, which you put right back on by eating an iced cupcake.' And Dr Stillman: 'even walking at moderate speed for a full hour uses only about 200 calories; no amount of exercising will reduce you if you over-eat.'

Professor Yudkin looks kindly upon exercise but says, nevertheless, that 'to dispose of a single cheese sandwich you would have to play squash for an hour. And to dispose of a good business lunch, you would have to play squash for eight hours.' At a press conference held by the Obesity Research Foundation in London in August 1982 Derek Miller of Queen Elizabeth College repeated the claim made in diet books that to get rid of the energy content of a hearty meal it would be necessary to walk up and down Ben Nevis.

The message was clear, for me. Fat people eat too much. Slim people do not hike up Britain's highest mountain after dinner, nor do they get on their bikes after eating a cupcake. The harm was in greed, not in sloth.

Diet books get their information from textbooks. A calorie as defined by a standard work of reference is:

A unit in which energy is measured. Technically, a calorie is the amount of heat necessary to raise the temperature of a gram of water one degree Centigrade. Food energy is measured in kilocalories.

(A kilocalorie is 1000 calories. But most people, nutritionists included, refer to a kilocalorie simply as a calorie.) Research on the energy value of food and of exercise started at the end of the nineteenth century. Nutrition textbooks now give calorie values of snack foods. So:

|  | *measure* | *calories* |
|---|---|---|
| Cupcake (chocolate, iced) | 2¾ inches diameter | 185 |
| Sandwiches: Ham | 1 sandwich | 280 |

It seems that Dr Tarnower favoured a large cupcake. (Ham and cheddar cheese have roughly the same calorie value.)

Other textbooks, on exercise physiology, give the calorie value of every kind of exercise for people of different weights (the more you weigh, the more energy you use up in any activity). Below are figures for a 'standard' 8 stone 8 woman and 11 stone man:

|  | *minutes* | *8 st 8 lb* *cals* | *11 st* *cals* |
|---|---|---|---|
| Cycling (leisure, 9.4 mph) | 30 | 168 | 213 |
| Squash | 60 | 714 | 916 |

It seems that Dr Tarnower was a fast cyclist. On the other hand, unless Professor Yudkin eats heroic sandwiches or plays a very leisurely game of squash, his figures are wildly wrong. However, his point can be made more modestly by proposing that a cheese sandwich (280 calories) takes an hour of walking off (270 calories for the 8 stone 8 woman, 342 calories for the 11 stone man). Dr John Garrow, in his book *Treat Obesity Seriously*, estimates that the fabled run of Pheidippides, the original marathon run to announce the victory of the Greeks over the Persians, cost him about 2500 calories. In the legend, Pheidippides died on arrival.

## Calorie counting

Leaving exercise aside, I turned to the diet books that claimed that I could, by means of self-denial and their regime, lose 10 pounds or more a week. In any case, I was a dieting expert. I believed the diet books; they worked. My problem was that after I stopped the diet I regained the weight I had lost. The fault, I was sure, was mine. I was a backslider. I was greedy.

What should I weigh? My ideal related to the tables of 'desirable body weight for men' published in books and magazines, and screwed on weighing-machines. These tables were devised by an American, Louis Dublin, for the Metropolitan Life Insurance Company. Dublin later decided to categorise people into arbitrary large-, medium- and small-frame sizes.

According to the tables my 'desirable' body weight, at slightly over 5 foot 11½ inches and wearing indoor clothing, is:

| Height | Small | Frame Medium | Large |
|--------|-------|--------|-------|
| | pounds | pounds | pounds |
| 5 foot 11 | 144-154 | 150-165 | 159-179 |
| 6 foot | 148-158 | 154-170 | 164-184 |

These 'desirable weights' varied from a little less than my heaviest weight ever to my lightest: nearly 3 stone. The range for a woman of average height is nearly 2 stone. I decided privately that 'large frame' was polite for 'fat' and that the tables were nonsense. Nor, in honest moments, did I go in for the idea that I had heavy bones. Nevertheless, the tables retained their fascination. I had a dream; I aspired to the bottom of the 'small-frame' scale. I had no idea of what the weight of my own body should be. I wanted to reduce myself to a statistic.

How much should I eat? Diet books rely on textbooks listing recommended energy intake and these books in turn determine how much energy in the form of food should be produced and supplied to national and international populations. There is general agreement about human energy requirements. The US Government recommends that the energy intake of a 'standard' man of 11 stone and 5 foot 10 inches tall who engages in 'light activity' should be:

| Age | Daily calorie intake range |
|-----|--------|
| 19-22 | 2500-3300 |
| 23-50 | 2300-3100 |
| 51-75 | 2000-2800 |
| 76+ | 1650-2450 |

'Light activity' is defined as 'sleep or lie down for eight hours a day, sit for seven hours, stand for five, walk for two, and spend two hours a day in light physical activity', which summed me up well enough, in those days. 'For adults, it is believed that an 800 calorie range covers most individuals,' says one textbook. The energy requirements of the standard woman weighing 8 stone 8 pounds and 5 foot 4 tall are 1200 calories a day at the lowest end of the scale for a 76+-year-old and 2500 calories a day at the top end of the scale for a 19- to 22-year-old.

The bigger you are, the more energy you need. And the older you are, the less energy you need, because people tend to slow down as they get older.

This is why diet books tell you to cut down your energy intake from food to 1500 calories a day or less. Audrey Eyton, in *The F-Plan Diet*, says: 'Allow yourself 1500 calories daily if you are male, of at least medium height, and more than half a stone overweight .... Allow yourself 1000 calories daily if you are female and less than one stone overweight.'

Dr Tarnower says, 'The Scarsdale Medical Diet averages 1000 calories or less a day.' Dr Stillman is very stern. 'You may falsify a calorie total on paper, but your body adds correctly and will turn into fat any extra calories that you omit by fake mathematics.' At one point he recommends a lettuce, lean meat and hard-boiled egg diet totalling 354 calories a day. Another Stillman diet, for the fainter-hearted, is the 'Six Meals-A-Day Nibbler Diet'. Of this he says, 'Whereas 900 to 1000 calories is the usual number allowed on a calorie-counting diet the nibbler diet allows you 1200 to 1800 calories a day.' This calorific cornucopia is against Dr Stillman's nature. 'For desirable quick weight loss,' he goes on, 'start with 900 to 1200 calories daily and then you may increase after you've learned control.'

Diet doctors tend to be stern. Dr Arnold Fox devised *The Beverly Hills Medical Diet* (BHMD; it has nothing to do with Judy Mazel's regime). 'Lose 10 pounds in 14 days! Enjoy potatoes, pasta and other forbidden foods,' promises the front cover. But when Dr Fox comes to define what he calls 'freedom with responsibility' he says, 'You are permitted to mix different recipes and to redesign the menus according to your personal preferences—provided you don't exceed the 1200 calorie limit.' And he goes on: 'Consult the BHMD calorie chart to determine the calorie count of each recipe.'

'The fewer calories you consume, the more quickly you will lose weight—within limits,' writes Professor Yudkin, and 'A daily 1000 calories is normally recommended as the safe low-calorie limit.' Whether diet books favour fibre (Eyton), protein (Stillman, Tarnower), carbohydrate (Fox) or oppose carbohydrate (Yudkin) the story is the same: lose weight by cutting calories, usually to 1000 to 1500 a day.

Dieters feel that their fat is their fault and that they are fat because they eat too much. Dieting is fuelled by guilt and self-disgust. Many dieters feel that the most conspicuous and inescapable evidence of their general failure to manage themselves and their world is their fat. Fat people believe that they are unfit and unhealthy. Hatred of being fat, and fear of becoming fat, are demoralising and disturbing to the point, for many dieters, of affecting their sanity. I know: I was there. I was alienated from my body; it was out of my control. Cyril Connolly wrote, 'Imprisoned in every fat man, a thin one is wildly signalling to be let out.' The thin being has been taken over; surrounded in the most literal way, by the alien, fat being.

Clearly, from what I had read, exercise could do little for me. The British Code of Advertising Practice on slimming aids confirms this view:

> A diet is the only practicable self-treatment for achieving a reduction in excess fat . . . . Claims, whether direct or indirect, that weight loss can be achieved by any other means are not acceptable.

But what to do? I dieted, I lost weight, I regained the weight, I grew fat. I was my own enemy.


### Could it be greed?

Something that vaguely puzzled me at the time was that I didn't think I was eating all that much. 'Self-deceit!' say the diet doctors. An acquaintance of mine, a doctor who is a nutritionist with a busy private practice of fat patients who want to be thin, regards them as naughty children who need discipline: firm instructions, an ordered regime. Otherwise, he tells me, they'll always cheat. The usual fable of the health farm is of the delinquent fatties who lure their fellows in obesity over the perimeter at dead of night for a gastronomic orgy at the local hotel.

Did I raid the refrigerator at night more often than other people? Were my portions larger, my meals bigger? Was I addicted to snacks? Diet books even include stories of people who go on sleep-walking binges. Could that be me? I watched friends and colleagues as we ate. They tucked in; they were not fat. I ate, feelings of self-disgust alternating with feelings of 'to hell with it'; I was fat. Was I really eating more than they were? Did they raid the refrigerator? Did they buy chocolate bars on the way home? These are questions you don't ask. But why was I never rewarded by my bouts of dieting? The great card-sharp in the sky seemed to have stacked the deck against me.

Some people do, indeed, eat compulsively, and thereby become obese. I had the impression that the average fat person was a big eater—why else should people get fat?—and that gargantuan appetite led to obesity. For a man, the images are of two kings, Henry VIII and Edward VII: the one throwing gnawed haunches of venison over his shoulder; the other gobbling breakfasts of partridge pie, cold mutton, truffles, a dozen plover's eggs and kedgeree, washed down with a pint of claret.

While not having such a regal appetite, I assumed that my problem was greed. But my assumption was contradicted by the measurement of the energy equivalent of fat on which all diet books base their calculations. Diet books start from the position that the energy equivalent of a pound of fat is 3500 calories (or, to use the exact term, 'kcal'). Thus, Audrey Eyton, in *The F-Plan Diet*, instancing a woman whose normal energy requirement is 2000 calories a day:

If we were to put you on a slimming diet providing you with 1500 calories a day, you would be 500 calories short of your requirement and these would have to be taken from your body fat. It has been scientifically estimated that a pound of your own body fat provides approximately 3500 calories. So during a week you would be likely to shed one pound of surplus fat.

And, by the same calculation, anyone who not only abandons the F-Plan but also consumes 500 calories too many will gain 1 pound of surplus fat every week.

John Durnin, Professor of Physiology at the University of Glasgow, has told me that this calculation is inaccurate. It is based on laboratory experiments made 100 years ago which do not take account of the biochemistry within the human body. He says that

> losing one pound of fat would result in a net energy deficit nearer 3000 kcal. More important, because the mechanical and biochemical efficiency of depositing adipose [fatty] tissue is relatively inefficient, you need about 4500 kcal to lay down one pound of fat in the body.

## A tangerine too many

Allowing for Professor Durnin's correction, a reminder that human chemistry is more subtle than the chemistry conducted in laboratories on inert material, then many of us would indeed be gross. An extra 4500 calories a week is just under 650 calories a day. According to Dr Fox's BHMD Diet, 650 calories may be composed of:

| | |
|---|---|
| Hamburger, broiled, regular, 3 oz | 245 |
| Potato crisps, 2 in diameter, 10 crisps | 115 |
| Beer, 12 fl oz (2) | 300 |

Or, from a standard textbook:

| | |
|---|---|
| Chocolate, plain (3.5 oz) | 525 |
| Peanuts, salted (1 oz) | 143 |

Or, from Audrey Eyton's *F-Plan Calorie and Fibre Chart*:

| | |
|---|---:|
| Cake, fruit, plain, average slice (2) | 400 |
| Biscuit, digestive wheatmeal (4) | 280 |

So, according to these figures, and on the diet books' arithmetic, a couple of snacks a day over the odds in a cafe, bar or at home will result in the consumption of food with an energy content of 650 calories or more.

In this case, if the diet books are to be believed, anyone who eats this quantity of food surplus to their daily requirements will gain a pound of fat a week, which is to say over 50 pounds a year or over 500 every ten years.

I seemed to gain about 12 pounds a year. It was difficult to be precise, since, when not on a diet, I was usually making up weight lost from the previous diet.

The weekly equivalent of 12 pounds a year is near enough 4 ounces. Given that these 4 ounces are fat, the caloric equivalent—allowing for Professor Durnin's correction of the textbook figures—is 1100 a week, or 160 a day, extra to my requirement.

So, if my problem was, indeed, that I was eating 160 calories a day too many each day the answer should be simple. According to the diet books, I should be able to maintain a steady weight by every day saying 'no' to any of the following, give or take the odd calorie:

| | | |
|---|---|---|
| Sweet biscuits, 1 oz (2) | 160-170 | (*Which?*) |
| Yogurt, low-fat, hazelnut, 5.3 oz | 160 | (Eyton) |
| Martini | 150 | (Stillman) |
| Gingerbread, 2×2×2 in (1) | 180 | (Tarnower) |
| Wine, dessert (4 oz glass) | 160 | (Fox) |

It is difficult to wrap the brain around the notion that one glass of wine (or one pint of beer) over the odds is evidence of greed. Furthermore, a weight gain of 12 pounds a year is 120 pounds a decade, an increase that would take me from an initial post-diet weight of 11 stone 7 pounds, say, to 20 stone. That, of course, was what I feared, the fate to which I believed I was doomed, unless I dieted. British weighing-machines often stop at 18 stone. The thought of going off the scale was a waking nightmare.

The fact is, though, that people who gain fat do not do so at anything like the rate of 120 pounds a year. A more typical rate of increase, for the man or woman who in time becomes over-fat, and one of the 65 per cent of British women or 30 per cent of British men who (according to the Royal College of Physicians in 1983) try to lose weight each year, would not be 120 pounds a decade but perhaps 30 pounds. This would change the slim young woman aged 20 weighing 8 stone into a woman aged 25 weighing just over 9 stone and into one of 30 weighing over 10 stone who will be worrying about her weight. Likewise, a man who between the ages of 20 and 30 increased from 11 stone to over 13 stone would metamorphose from being slim to being decidedly overweight and liable to worry about becoming obese in the next decade. (These figures assume sedentary women and men of average height; taller people might gain rather more weight proportionately from a heavier initial weight.)

The energy equivalent of a gain of 30 pounds of fat in a decade is 40 calories of energy from food a day. Forty calories a day? The diet books count them:

| | | |
|---|---|---|
| Potato crisps, 2 in diameter, (4) | 46 | (Fox) |
| Tangerine, raw, 2½ in diameter | 40 | (Tarnower) |
| Butter, 1 pat | 50 | (Stillman) |
| Pickle, sweet, 1 oz (1 rounded tbsp) | 40 | (Eyton) |
| Tomatoes, fried, 2 oz | 40-50 | (*Which?*) |

Most diet books recommend calorie control. Theirs is a world where the dieter is invited to measure potato crisps with a ruler and to believe that eating four more than the body's requirements will lead to a weight gain of 30 pounds in a decade (to be exact, close to 35 pounds according to Dr Fox's calculations, assuming that the crisps are round and not elliptical). And eating three less than requirement —a difference of seven crisps—will lead to a weight loss of 30 pounds in a decade.

No diet book has ever made such a claim, because it is absurd. But there it is: the arithmetic, supposedly based on science, proposes that one tangerine too many, every day, is the path to obesity. Can such a notion possibly be true?

### Three crisps too few

Consider the arithmetic for the person who eats three crisps too few each day. (This amounts to a 2-ounce packet of crisps too many or too few once a week.) The consequent and apparently inexorable weight loss would mean that the slim young woman of 9 stone aged 20 would weigh 2 stone 8 pounds aged 50. If she underdid it not by three but by four crisps a day, by the age of 50 she would have disappeared altogether.

Consider a different case: the person who does eat or drink quite a lot too much. Take, say, the man who puts away 3 pints of beer and a couple of packets of peanuts a day, on top of eating and drinking enough for his body's needs. (If that is greed, there is a lot of it about.) This extra intake, with a pint of bitter at 175 calories and peanuts at 300 calories a 50-gram packet, is 1125 calories a day. At that rate, the 4500 calories equals 1 pound of fat equation implies that this moderate drinker would gain about 8 pounds a month, or just under 100 pounds every year.

Professor Durnin cites the case of William Campbell, the Scot who died aged 22 in 1878 having established the United Kingdom record for obesity, at 341 kg. 'We can estimate,' says Durnin:

> that in his 22 years he acquired fat representing an excess over intake of about 1¾ million kcal. If we now calculate what average daily excess would be required to achieve his record-breaking weight in 22 years, the answer comes to 218 kcal a day.

And, Durnin goes on to point out, well aware that his fellow-Scots are known to drink a pint or two a day and even eat the odd peanut: 'Differences of this magnitude, of 200 kcal, are frequently found between measurements of the average daily intake and the energy expenditure of the individual.' In which case, what can overweight have to do with greed?

In my dieting days, I never did the sums necessary to show that the reasoning of the diet books advocating calorie control was preposterous. Although calorie counting did strike me as obsessive to the point of being deranged, I took the basic propositions of the books on trust. After all, every diet I went on worked. They succeeded. I failed.

I was also concerned about my health. The diet books have ways of keeping the dieter obedient. Dr Stillman has a chapter entitled 'Facts to Help "Scare" the Fat off You'. He quotes Brillat-Savarin. 'Well, go ahead and eat and grow fat,' the French gourmet said. 'Become ugly, heavy, have asthmatic attacks and die choked by your own fat.' Or, according to Stillman, Tarnower, and indeed *Which? Way to Slim*, suffer or die from diabetes, gall-stones, arthritis, strokes, heart disease. 'If you're 10 per cent overweight,' says Stillman 'you'll lose seven years of living. In effect you will have committed suicide at 63.' I did not want to suffer or die prematurely. What was the matter with me? Could I be saved?

### Fat people eat less

John Garrow is often cited as the leading authority on obesity in England. He wrote in 1974 that there is 'no evidence of any relationship between energy intake and body weight in man'. In 1977 at a congress on obesity he said that no evidence had been found 'that obese people ate more than thin ones. The cause of obesity is astonishingly difficult to pin down.' I asked Dr Garrow if any evidence had emerged since 1977 to show that fat people ate more than thin people. He said no.

In 1974 Professor Durnin, in a study made in Glasgow, found that fat girls did not eat more than thin girls: they ate less than thin girls. Durnin also made two studies of 14-year-old boys and girls, in 1964 and 1971. Calorie intake had fallen by 180 to 250 calories a day during the seven years. In 1971 the boys who were eating less were fatter than the 1964 boys. (Girls stayed much the same.) Nutritionist Alison Paul and others undertook a variation of this study in 1982 and discovered that today's teenagers eat fewer calories than their parents and, indeed, eat 300 to 500 calories a day less than is recommended by the World Health Organisation. But nevertheless they tend to be overweight.

In 1979 Professor Harry Keen reported on a study of links between what and how much people eat and diabetes. As part of his study he measured the amount of food people ate, and their degree of fatness, in three population samples: 961 employees of Beechams Foods; 1005 employees of the Greater London Council; and 1488 middle-aged male civil servants. What he found, to his surprise, was 'highly significant inverse correlations between food energy intake and adiposity (degree of fatness), a relation found in both sexes and in all three population samples.'

That is to say, the fatter people were eating less than the thinner people. This applied to both men and women and to all the groups studied. Keen eliminated people who were slimming from his analysis; this did not affect his results. He considered the possibility that the fatter people were underestimating how much they were eating; but such self-deception is only known among some obese people, and Keen's study was of people who did not see themselves as having a weight problem. Also, Keen's discovery that thinner people ate more and that fatter people ate less applied right across the range of thinness and fatness, not just to those people who were most overweight. As was to be expected, Keen found that people got fatter as they got older; but the rule that fatter people ate less and thinner people ate more applied to all ages.

The Royal College of Physicians, commenting in their 1983 report on obesity on surveys of British men and women done in the last 50 years, states: 'There now seems little doubt that there is a general trend for both men and women to become heavier and presumably fatter, this change being particularly evident in young adults.'

As judged by the 1981 census, the proportion of British people carrying excess weight is about a quarter of men and women in their 20s and just under a half of men and women over the age of 40. The figures are

| Age | Men | Women |
|---|---|---|
| | (Percentage with excess weight) | |
| 16–19 | 15 | 15 |
| 20–24 | 22 | 23 |
| 25–29 | 29 | 20 |
| 30–39 | 40 | 25 |
| 40–49 | 52 | 38 |
| 50–59 | 49 | 47 |
| 60–65 | 54 | 50 |
| Total | 39 | 32 |

The estimated amount of body fat has also risen steadily in the last 20 years.

But the *National Food Survey*, an official publication, shows that the amount of energy consumed from food has steadily dropped in the last 20 years. In 1960 the British people were consuming 2628 calories a day from food. In 1981 the figure had dropped to 2210: a fall of 19 per cent. The figures for recent years are

| 1960 | 1965 | 1970 | 1975 | 1979 | 1980 | 1981 |
|---|---|---|---|---|---|---|
| 2628 | 2590 | 2560 | 2290 | 2250 | 2230 | 2210 |

These figures probably exaggerate the drop in energy intake from food because they do not take into account food eaten outside the home; and consumption of snack food has risen in the 1970s. The Ministry of Agriculture compiles statistics of food imported and produced in Britain before it is processed. These figures do not allow for the waste of food in manufacture and thereafter, but they do include food eaten outside the home. They show that consumption of refined sugar reached a peak in 1977 and that alcohol consumption is continuing to rise; and that overall there was a drop of 222 calories a day energy from food consumed between 1960 and 1981.

We are getting fatter while eating less. Professor Peter Wood of Stanford University confirms that the same is true in the USA and adds, referring to findings from the USA, Britain and other Western countries, 'These facts relate to an interesting finding from several large population studies; generally speaking fatter people eat less than thinner people.'

But if over-eating is not the cause of obesity, so that the very word 'obese' (derived from *ob*—'over' and *edere*—'to eat') is based on a misconception, what makes people fat? If not gluttony, then what? The answer seemed to lie in a word not much mentioned in the diet books but which has crept into many women's magazine features lately: 'metabolism'. The Obesity Research Foundation says:

> The ability of some people to eat what they like and not gain weight is the constant envy of the obese. It would seem that the lean and the obese are metabolically different, and the explanation of the difference is an urgent challenge to science.

My granny used to say that fat people had something wrong with their glands; I thought this was a homely way of saying, as is often said now, that fat people have 'a low metabolism' or, more correctly, 'a low metabolic rate'. Was this my doom? Had the great double-dealer in the sky given me an unwinnable hand? Should fat people not be scorned as greedy, but pitied as helpless?

### Eating like a bird and like a horse

The notion that fat people are lumbered with a low metabolism has been popularised by Dr Robert C Atkins, whose *Diet Revolution*, *Super-Energy Diet* and *Nutrition Breakthrough* have sold a total of twelve million books, worldwide. Dr Atkins is as enthusiastic about his books as Dr Stillman and Dr Tarnower were about theirs. He maintains that

Failure to lose weight on a diet low in both calories and carbohydrates is strong evidence of a metabolic imbalance ... variations in metabolic responses are important factors in obesity, and any physician should know that he will be seeing many cases of impaired response.

Metabolism can be defined as 'the sum total of all the chemical reactions that go on in living cells'. Metabolic rate is the speed at which the body uses energy which it needs for the constant process of replacing and renewing cells in all its parts while asleep and at rest; for the digestion of food; and for activity. Most people use most energy not for activity but for the workings of their vital organs—the brain, heart, liver and kidneys especially. Put simply, metabolic rate is the speed at which our bodies work.

It is commonplace, nowadays, for people to describe themselves as having either (luckily) a 'high metabolism' or (unluckily) a 'low metabolism'. The assumption is that we are stuck with the metabolic rate with which we are born. The fault is not in ourselves—in our sloth, or greed, or both—but in our genes. (Indeed, people more sophisticated than my gran use 'genes' rather than 'glands' as an excuse for obesity.)

Interestingly, this determinist proposition is similar to the now discredited theory that we are stuck with the intelligence (IQ) with which we are born. It takes away a sense of personal responsibility for our physical shape and blames the Almighty, or heredity. In my case, my father is over-fat, whereas his father was lean; so I half-believed that when the chromosomal dice were cast I got the low metabolic numbers. I was a slow burner; I was one of those who gained weight as soon as I 'looked at a bun', because I had a low metabolism. My friends and colleagues who ate heartily but evidently gained no weight had a high metabolism.

One analogy for metabolism is engine capacity. Thus, a middle-aged woman may have a Mini-Minor capacity and so eat 'like a bird' and yet be plump; whereas a young man with a Range-Rover capacity can 'eat like a horse' and yet stay lean. And, just as Mini-Minors do not turn into Range-Rovers, nor birds into horses, the inference is that metabolic rate is inborn. Analogies always carry inferences.

Another analogy often used for human metabolism is the central heating system. Hence the concept of the 'appestat'. Yudkin says: 'You could more or less describe the appestat as the part of the brain that controls how much we eat in the same way that a thermostat controls temperature.' But 'if you are overweight, you don't stop wanting to eat when you've had enough. So obviously something has gone wrong with your appestat.' The thermostat that controls the temperature of my bath-water is set at 175°F, just as the thermostatic mechanism that controls the temperature of my body is set at 98.4°F.

If I now go to my water-heater and turn the thermostat up to 185°F, I shall quite soon become too hot, because the heater is also part of my central heating system. If the heater's thermostat jammed at 185°F, it would be too high and would have gone wrong. With this analogy in mind, a number of scientists, aware that fat people do not characteristically eat more than thin people, have proposed the 'set-point' theory. This supposes that people who tend to obesity suffer from a condition in which the mechanism that regulates their body weight is set too high.

### Born to be fat?

A champion of 'set-point' theory is Professor Richard Keesey of the University of Wisconsin. Keesey works with rats. He says:

> Laboratory animals, like human beings, appear to regulate body weight around a stable level or set-point. If their weight is reduced by restricting their calorie intake, rats rapidly restore body weight to the level of nonrestricted controls when allowed to feed freely . . . Thus, as in man, the stability and the vigorous defence of its body weight by the rat suggest the presence of a set-point regulator.

That is to say, I was born to be fat. The implication of this ingenious theory is that my weight, when I was dieting, was never meant to fluctuate; that it went down—and then up—because I dieted; and that if I left well alone and ate what I wanted, my weight would stop at some point, and stay steady at that 'set' point.

In *The Dieter's Dilemma* Dr William Bennett and Joel Gurin have popularised set-point theory. They say:

> Some individuals come with a high setting, others with a low one. Some are therefore naturally fat and others thin. Going on a diet is an attempt to overpower the body's set-point; it is not a fair contest. The set-point is a tireless opponent.

'Your setting,' they go on, 'is the weight you normally maintain, give or take a few points, when you are not thinking about it.'

'The set-point theory is, admittedly, somewhat fatalistic,' say Bennett and Gurin. But it does have charm. It suggests that the dieter's problem is not becoming fat but refusing to accept that she or he is designed by nature to be fat. Love it! 'The obsessive drive to be thin serves no real purpose, except to funnel large amounts of money into the diet industry,' they say. And: 'The prejudice against fatness is cruel, destructive, and unfair.' They find support from the 'Fat is Beautiful' movement in the USA and also from Susie Orbach, whose book *Fat is a Feminist Issue* quite rightly sees tyranny in the pressure put on women to become super slim.

Was there, then, truth in what my granny told me? Was I born to be fat?

Set-point theory cannot explain why the average body fat content of the British adult population has increased by 10 per cent in the last 40 years. (Statistics from the USA are similar.) Set-point theory, the darling of many writers in America, falls to the ground. It has to be far-fetched. In any case, is it true that 'most of us remain on essentially the same body weight', as set-point theory proposes?

No, it isn't. Set-point theory was discredited before many people had heard of it, let alone believed it. In 1974 a survey of long-stay prisoners in Wormwood Scrubs, whose body weight was measured in the eight years between 1965 and 1972, was published in a book by Dr John Garrow, who explained:

> It may be that long-stay prisoners are not typical of the general population, but on general grounds one might expect that their weight would be more stable than that of the population at liberty; their way of life is more like that of laboratory animals which show great stability of body weight.

And the results of the routine weighing of these prisoners? 'On average their weight varied over a range of 7.5 kg (16.6 pounds) during a period of seven years.'

Garrow supported his findings by quoting studies of more than 1000 people in Wales over four years, which showed weight deviations of over 20 pounds; and of the community of Framingham in the USA in which 'on average, both men and women fluctuated by 10 kg (22 pounds) over 18 years.'

So much for set-point theory. Man is not a rat. In 1976, my last year of dieting, I was not aware of set-point theory, but I was no closer than its champions have ever been to finding out why I got fat. If the reason wasn't sloth, and wasn't greed, and wasn't genes, what could it be?

### Exercise: the key?

In his *Super-Energy Diet* Dr Atkins calls one chapter 'If You Are Not Getting Results'. Addressed to hopeless cases, it includes a tip which sounds the most loony but harmless remedy for the overweight ever proposed. 'A surefire trick if you can afford it,' he says, is to 'go to Europe'. How could this help me? I live in Europe. But Dr Atkins perseveres:

> For some strange reason, as yet unexplained, a trip to Europe always seems to help with weight reduction. It may be something in the soil .... The best results seem to be achieved in Mediterranean countries: Spain, Greece, Italy, or the south of France.

In summer 1979 I had not read Dr Atkins, and I had abandoned dieting, having decided that I'd rather get fat than go mad. I went on holiday to Greece for a month to a tiny island in the Cyclades. When I left England, I weighed a flabby 12 stone 12. When I returned I was down 10 pounds at 12 stone 2. I have kept this weight ever since, give or take a few pounds, while eating and drinking whatever I want. For the first time my weight has been stable.

What had happened in Greece? Its clean air had given me a good appetite, and this book does not propose that eating makes you thin.

Nor was the reason that I was taking more exercise than usual. The reverse was true—for the previous autumn I had started to jog. I had been in Hyde Park, watching the first *Sunday Times* National Fun Run. The exaltation of the runners, some almost twice my age, was an inspiration—not to start running to lose weight, but to join in running, to participate. Watching the runners, and reflecting on an imminent fortieth birthday, I came to three conclusions: I was a spectator of, not a participant in, my own life; there are no easy ways out, and nothing worthwhile is easy; and if I didn't start then, I never would.

So I started to jog. By the next summer I was doing gentle 4½-mile runs and sometimes covered 20 miles in a week. Then came the Greek holiday, during which I enjoyed walking, and some swimming, and a sense of well-being earned by my new fitness that I'd never experienced before as an adult. But I took no more, and probably less, exercise on that holiday than in the previous months. Afterwards I regarded the weight loss as an enigma.

Since then, running has become part of my life. I've lost no more weight, but I have changed shape. And talking with many people about the effect of exercise on weight and fat I have found plenty who, like me, started running when 10 to 30 pounds overweight, lost weight, lost fat, and now eat and drink what they like. It was when I realised that I would never again have to diet that I started the research for this book.

CHAPTER TWO

# *Dieting Makes You Fat*

The Holy Grail of Western medicine is a safe and comfortable way to lose excessive body fat. This fruitless search has been the basis of an almost endless array of 'reducing diets' that have tantalised the fat folks and enriched the publishers and the medical businessmen. The reducing diets have been disappointing—some would say, a medical disaster.

GEORGE MANN
*New England Journal of Medicine*

It was not through statements that we learned how to breathe, swallow, see, circulate the blood, digest food, or resist diseases. Yet these things are performed by the most complex and marvellous processes which no amount of booklearning and technical skill can reproduce. But we have been taught to neglect, despise and violate our bodies, and to put all our faith in our brains. As a consequence, we are at war within ourselves—the brain desiring things which the body does not want, and the body desiring things which the brain does not allow; the brain giving directions which the body will not follow, and the body giving impulses which the brain cannot understand.

ALAN WATTS
*The Wisdom of Insecurity*

## *The big slow down*

A successful diet book is liable to sell millions of copies worldwide. People who want to lose weight do not try to do so for fun. For many people, their desire to lose weight matters as much as anything else in their lives.

Dieters are entitled to expect that any writer of a diet book will have at least an elementary knowledge of the effects of dieting on the human body. As a rule, diet books are based on two assumptions about dieting. First, that diets do not affect the speed at which the body works—the metabolic rate. Second, that weight lost on a diet is all or almost all fat. 'When you are slimming you are really eating your own body—eating away the part of it you don't want, that surplus fat!' says Audrey Eyton in her *F-Plan Diet*.

It is a pity to single out Mrs Eyton, because her F-Plan recommends eating food rich in fibre, which is nourishing, whereas the foods recommended by other diet books are often debilitating or even dangerous. But she is typical of writers of diet books when she says, having made the '1 pound of body fat equals 3500 calories' calculation, that:

> Expected rate of fat loss has always been estimated simply by counting the calories consumed in the form of food, any food, and subtracting them from the number the body requires for energy. . . . With a daily deficit of 1000 calories you could expect to shed around two pounds a week.

But is it true that diets do not affect the speed at which the body works? No, it is not. Diets slow down the metabolic rate. And is it true that weight lost on diets is fat or almost all fat? No, it is not. Much of the weight lost on a diet is not fat; and any initial fast weight loss is not because of removal of fat.

These facts have been known for many years. Research into the effect of diets on the body started at the beginning of this century and has been repeated again and again. The silence of diet books on the effects of dieting on the body is so total, and the profits to be made from them are so large, that it is impossible to believe that all diet books are written in good faith. They lead readers to believe that when diets fail it is the dieter who is to blame. Of course they do; the writer of a diet book doesn't want the reader to doubt the book, and self-doubt helps diet book sales. In fact, diets fail because of what they do to the body of the dieter.

What happens to the body of a dieter depends to a considerable extent on the nature, severity and length of the diet, and also on the body composition, eating habits and way of life of the dieter.

First, any diet book that claims or suggests that an initial weight loss of 10 to 15 pounds a week is of fat is misleading the reader, as a simple calculation will show. The energy required to burn off a pound of body fat is 3000 calories (Professor Durnin's correct figure). It follows that the energy required to burn off 10 to 15 pounds of fat a week is 30,000 to 45,000 calories, or 4286 to 6429 calories a day. But diet regimes recommend cutting down by 500 to 1500 calories a day. There is thus no way that the initial fast weight loss, which dieters are led to believe is proof of success, can be of body fat. Simple mathematics prove the point.

(Some of the more reckless writers of diet books, usually those first published in the USA, suggest that the foods recommended on their regimes have a special fat-burning property in addition to their low-calorie value. These claims are nonsense; they have the same sort of relationship to nutrition as astrology does to astronomy.)

### Burning the glycogen

The body's first reaction to a diet regime is to draw on the energy that is immediately available in any emergency. This is not from fat, but from a substance in the body that you do not hear about in diet books: glycogen. Glycogen is a form of glucose (a carbohydrate), stored in solution with water in the muscles and in the body's most metabolically active vital organ, the liver. The body normally contains about 8 to 10 pounds of glycogen.

Glycogen burns very much faster than ordinary fat. A footballer playing hard in the sun or a marathon runner can lose up to 10 pounds, or even more, of glycogen and water in two or three hours. I myself have lost eight pounds running a half-marathon on a humid summer day. A special diet used by marathon runners (the so-called 'carbohydrate-bleeding' regime) consists of food specially designed to drain the glycogen stores, and loses about 6 pounds in three days. It is not a calorie-controlled diet: you can eat as much as you like of very high-protein foods such as meat, fish, eggs and cheese. (The runners then follow the 'bleeding' regime with 'carbohydrate-loading' for the three days before a marathon, in order to saturate their bodies with energy-giving carbohydrates.)

The effect is the same as the diet regimes of Dr Stillman and Dr Tarnower, which recommend high protein and low carbohydrate; and of Dr Atkins, which recommends high fat and low carbohydrate. It is these diets which drain the body's own carbohydrate store—glycogen—fastest. The body must have carbohydrate: the brain, for example, uses glucose released into the blood almost exclusively as a fuel and has practically no glucose store of its own.

Low-carbohydrate diets drain the body's glycogen stores in the first few days without touching the body's fat stores at all. Any diet regime that cuts calories by means of cutting sugars and starches—the carbohydrates—will have this effect. The Royal College of Physicians recognised the phenomenon in their 1983 report on obesity, stating of diet regimes that:

> The patient needs to know that short-term rapid weight losses with rigorous diets depend on losses of body water (with glycogen and protein) rather than on losses of body fat.

Low glycogen levels trigger the mechanism in the body that signals hunger. Food such as bread, spaghetti, cereals, beans and potatoes are satisfying not just because of their energy content but because they are rich in starch, a nutritious carbohydrate, that feeds the glycogen stores, raises the blood glucose level, and gives a sense of fullness and well-being.

By contrast, a runner on the 'carbohydrate-bleeding' regime eats lots of protein and, with a full stomach, loses weight and becomes ravenously, obsessively hungry, thinking of little else but food. This hunger has nothing to do with an empty stomach or a low energy intake, nor is it caused by loss of fat. The cause, and the cause of the weight loss, is exhaustion of the glycogen store. Exactly the same happens to dieters who cut down or cut out carbohydrates—starches and sugars. The surest way to get someone obsessed with food is to put them on a diet regime.

Glycogen loss leads to low blood-sugar levels. The result is a sense of weakness, depression, irritation, tiredness, and sometimes faintness and dizziness. Dieters will recognise the pattern.

At the same time as losing glycogen bound up with water, dieters also lose water from elsewhere in the body. It is possible to lose 7 pounds of water sweating it out all night in a Turkish bath; I once won a lose-weight contest that way. Boxers and jockeys dehydrate themselves so as to weigh in under a required weight. The human body contains 50 to 65 per cent water. Women's bodies contain less water than men's, because body fat contains only a small amount of water, and the average woman has more fat than the average man. For the same reason, a fat person's body contains less water than that of a lean person of the same weight. Almost half our body weight is water contained within the body's cells. Water is essential for the body's metabolic processes. The body adapts to a diet by reducing the water content inside and outside the body's cells.

## Fat people stay fat

In our minds we know the difference between going on a diet and being subjected to famine or starvation. But our bodies do not know the difference. When we go on a diet regime we activate the mechanisms in the body that protect us and preserve us in times of famine. And what does the body need to keep it going between times of famine? Fat. The more often someone diets, the more their body will protect the stores of fat.

The human body can adapt to circumstances. It can get used to very hot or very cold weather, or to high altitude. The body constantly adjusts to accommodate a person's way of life, preserving what that person needs, if necessary at the expense of what is not needed, or at least not used.

Once a dieter's body has adapted to the diet by releasing glycogen and shedding water, it will then tend to lose the tissue it needs least.

The protein loss referred to by the Royal College of Physicians (see p. 49) means loss of lean tissue, including muscle. Diet regimes also have the effect of wasting lean body tissue. If the diet is severe or takes the form of a fast, much or even most tissue lost will be lean body tissue, including muscle.

The body of a sedentary dieter will tend to lose lean tissue, muscle in particular, simply because a sedentary person does not need much muscle. The longer the dieter has been sedentary, the stronger the tendency for lean tissue to be lost. And the body of a fat dieter will seek to preserve fat, simply because it is accustomed to fat.

By contrast, the body of an active and relatively lean person, even if it has a large bulk of muscle, will tend to lose body fat, simply because the body has learned that the muscle is needed; it is being used all the time.

There comes a point, even in an almost inert person, at which the body will protect its lean tissue. But this switch takes some time. Doctors can devise diets for anyone which, with persistence, will lose far more fat than lean tissue. But the body's processes include what can be termed 'tissue memory'. After a time, interpreted as a crisis, the body will tend to rebuild itself in the form appropriate to the uses to which it is put.

Lean, active people who go on a diet—boxers and jockeys for example—lose weight efficiently, lose fat if they have any to lose, eat a lot after dieting to keep their bright fires burning, and tend to gain muscle, the body having adapted to their way of life. (Heavyweight boxers who go to fat do so because in training they may be so active that they can eat up to 7000 calories a day. Out of training they often continue to eat a great deal of food without being sufficiently active to consume the energy from it.)

Most dieters are not boxers or jockeys but are fat, inactive people. When fat inactive people diet, their bodies adapt to the diet not according to what they have in mind but according to their way of life. They tend to lose relatively more lean tissue, which is not needed on their life's voyage.

To sum up: dieting, of the type recommended in diet books, results in loss of glycogen, water and lean tissue from the body. And loss of glycogen causes the hunger, fatigue and depression that dieters experience. Dieting also slows the body down.


### Adapting to a diet

First of all, a dieter is likely to become less active without necessarily even noticing. You may sleep a little longer, walk up stairs less often, not feel like tackling an energetic task, find that the television programmes have suddenly become very good, or just spend more time sitting and musing. In these situations the dieter is often not aware that a pattern of inactivity is forming, the means whereby the body seeks to make do with less food.

Equally, a dieter may also be conscious of becoming less active—'I'm taking it easy, I'm on a diet'. The result may be a pleasant sense of restfulness or an unpleasant sense of lassitude. For the body, the results are the same.

Dieters do not normally take to their beds. During any but the most rigorous diet activity is not usually dramatically reduced. But a man might use 150 to 450 calories a day less on activity, depending on whether he was sedentary or fairly active; a woman maybe 100 to 300 less.

Also, the less food you eat, the less energy you need to digest it. A diet that cuts 500 calories a day needs about 50 calories a day less energy for digestion. It follows, therefore, that if a fairly active person cuts 500 calories a day, their body need not lose significant amounts of fat, or of any other body tissue. The body of a fairly active person can adapt to a moderate diet by becoming the body of a sedentary person.

In practice anyone on a mild diet, if they keep to it, will lose some weight and also some fat. But no one can lose a pound of fat a week by cutting 500 calories of food a day, or anything like that amount, unless they consciously compensate for the body's adaptation to the diet by becoming more active.

The reason why diet books specify an energy intake of 1000 calories a day from food for women and 1500 calories a day for men (or levels of this order) is because the body needs more energy than this for its basic, vital functions.

At rest, it is the vital organs that have most work to do. The brain accounts for about 20 per cent of the body's energy used at rest. The liver is even more active, accounting for about 27 per cent of the body's activity at rest. The contribution of various parts of the body to energy turnover are estimated to be as follows:

| | |
|---|---|
| Liver (and associated areas) | 27 per cent |
| Brain | 20 |
| Heart | 7 |
| Kidneys | 10 |
| Skeletal muscle | 18 |
| Remainder | 18 |

At rest, then, about 65 per cent of the energy the body needs is used by vital organs whose weight totals about 5 per cent of the body's weight. Of the remaining 35 per cent, some is used by body fat, which is not inert but, like the rest of the body, requires nourishment and constantly renews itself. Most of the remaining energy is used by muscle, which is more active than body fat. How much more active depends on the condition of the muscle. The little-used muscles of a sedentary person are relatively inactive at rest. Muscle regularly used, say by someone who exercises vigorously three or four times a week, is relatively active at all times, not just during exercise. This is because the stress of exercise breaks down muscle tissue, and the muscle then actively regenerates. During exercise, the energy used by muscle increases dramatically, by twenty, fifty or even a hundred times more than the amount used at rest, depending on the condition of the muscles and the intensity of the exercise.

A sedentary person's body uses most of its energy from food for its vital autonomous functions. About 20 per cent will be used for living: sedentary activities such as sitting down, talking, writing and thinking: and somewhat more energetic activities, such as standing, walking around the home and the office, light work, and holidays spent mostly on the beach. This of course is an outline of the life style of millions of people in the West.

As already mentioned, the process of digestion uses about 10 per cent of the calories from food. Thus 2500 calories eaten in a day require 250 for digestion; 1500 calories require 150.

So a fair estimate of the energy needs of a sedentary person can be produced, allowing 20 per cent above the basic level for living and another 10 per cent for digestion. The term energy balance signifies the balance between energy taken in from food and from oxygen, and energy used by the body in all its activity. A sedentary man of average fat and weight (11 stone) will be in energy balance, and will therefore tend to stay the same weight, at about 2200 calories a day. An average woman (8 stone 8 pounds) will be in balance at about 1600 calories a day. In these examples energy taken in and used will be as follows:

|  | | Calories | | |
| --- | --- | --- | --- | --- |
|  | Rest | Digestion | Living | Total |
| Man (11 st) | 1700 | 200 | 300 | 2200 |
| Woman (8 st 8 lb) | 1250 | 150 | 200 | 1600 |

These figures are well below those recommended by the World Health Organisation for people described as 'fairly active', meaning people who walk around for quite a lot of the day, such as teachers and housewives who do their own household tasks and who also engage in regular light recreation such as gardening or golf at weekends. For these people, who take some trouble not to be sedentary, the WHO figures are:

|  | Total calories |
| --- | --- |
| Man (11 st) | 2940 |
| Woman (8 st 8 lb) | 2000 |

The energy required by the fairly active person for all activity, including digestion, is roughly half as much again as that required by the body at rest. But for fairly active as well as sedentary people the energy the body requires when asleep and at rest is much greater than that required for activity.

On a diet, the body of a fairly active person can thus accommodate a drop of a few hundred calories by becoming much less active. But the body of a sedentary person does not have so much room for manoeuvre. And in any case, diet regimes usually stipulate 1000 to 1500 calories a day or less.

How does the body accommodate such a sharp cut? The diet book theory, which might seem common sense, is that the body has no option but to lose fat. But in fact the body has many other options. And it not only takes these options so as to protect the storehouse of fat, by losing glycogen, water and lean tissue and by slowing down its waking activity. It also slows down its vital functions. The dieter's metabolic rate, like that of anyone who fasts or who is starving, slows down to adapt to the new situation.

The diet books have ignored the scientific studies of this phenomenon, although these are well known to specialists in obesity and energy balance. The fact that human metabolism is not static but dynamic, and is depressed by dieting, is such vital knowledge that it is worth going into some detail in describing the studies that have proved the point.

## Dieting slows you down

People who believe that dieting works have often said to me, 'but nobody ever got fat in a concentration camp'. This macabre fact is presented in support of the idea that what amounts to the voluntary semi-starvation of dieting will reduce overweight people to some point short of emaciation. Likewise, images of skeletal people on hunger strike or of the victims of famine remain in the minds of Westerners who regard themselves as well fed as evidence that dieting works.

Dr Marian Apfelbaum, of the Bichat Hospital in Paris, investigated what happened to the people of the Warsaw Ghetto during the two years of famine in the Second World War. It is known that the average daily calorie intake was between 700 and 800: roughly 1700 calories a day less than would have been consumed before the war.

It is safe to assume that the average weight of body fat (also known as 'adipose tissue') in an adult is about 30 pounds, representing roughly 100,000 calories. A deficit of 1700 calories a day for two years amounts to a total deficit of 1,000,000 calories, in round figures: 'approximately ten times the equivalent in energy of the adipose stores', as Apfelbaum says. What, then, happened to the remaining deficit of 900,000 calories?

A less extreme but better documented case is of 700 Swiss whose calorie intake was measured between 1942 and 1946. In 1942 the average intake was 2400 calories a day, as it was in 1946. In the intervening years, food restrictions forced the intake down to 2100 calories a day; then 2000, then 1850. The accumulated deficit, taking 2400 calories a day as the norm, was 600,000 calories per person. But the average weight loss for the whole period was 20 pounds a person which, measured as body fat, amounts to 60,000 calories. What happened to the remaining 540,000 calories?

Apfelbaum reviewed these cases of forced restriction of food because he was concerned with:

> The problem of an obese person who loses weight on a restricted diet but then stops. Physicians in the past have tended to say that such a patient must be a liar, because they considered that energy expenditure was not influenced by energy intake. I think they were wrong.

And he concluded: 'There is a wealth of evidence showing that there is a reduction in energy expenditure with restricted diet.' That is to say, dieting slows down the metabolic rate.

The classic experiments on the physiology of dieting were

carried out in the USA by F G Benedict in 1919 and by Ancel Keys in 1945. Benedict put thirty-four student volunteers on a diet first of 2100, then of 1500 calories a day: as healthy young men their normal requirement was 3100 calories. The goal of the experiment was to achieve a weight loss of 10 per cent, which took 60 days. But their metabolic rate declined to a greater extent than this loss of body weight could account for: by 18 per cent.

Keys' project was more ambitious. He restricted thirty-six volunteers to a diet of 1570 calories a day but for a longer period: 24 weeks. The volunteers were highly motivated, being conscientious objectors who felt it appropriate to deprive themselves. At the end of 24 weeks their weight had on average declined by 24 per cent. But their metabolic rate at rest had declined by 39 per cent.

The outward signs of this loss of vitality were lethargy and apathy. The young men lost interest in themselves, in each other, in sex and in visitors. They stopped spontaneous play and avoided work. Two had mental breakdowns. All became obsessed with food.

Some studies, including one recently made by Dr John Garrow and co-workers of nineteen very obese women who lost an average of 66 pounds in a year by means of jaw-wiring, have shown a drop in resting metabolic rate matched by weight loss. But studies of people on restricted diets in less extreme circumstances, corresponding to the situation of all but the most obese dieters, consistently support the findings of Benedict and Keys: the drop in metabolic rate outmatches the drop in weight.

George Bray, Professor of Medicine at UCLA, put six overweight women on a diet of 450 calories for 24 days. He reported in *The Lancet* that their weight dropped by an average of 22 pounds, a drop of 7 per cent. But their energy expenditure dropped by 15 per cent.

Derek Miller of Queen Elizabeth College, London, Audrey Eyton's nutritional adviser, is a campaigner against the notion that, as he puts it, obesity is caused by 'either or both of the deadly sins, gluttony and sloth'. He is clear that 'energy intake and expenditure influence each other'.

Like Apfelbaum, Miller contradicts the notion that dieters who say that they eat little are lying. He took thirty veteran dieters from slimming clubs to Ragdale Hall, an isolated country house. Their luggage was searched, their car keys taken away, and they were fed a diet supplying the same number of calories as Benedict and Keys gave their young male volunteers: 1500 a day. Miller's regime lasted for three weeks. The metabolic rate of these seasoned dieters was so low that 'although 19 subjects lost weight, nine maintained within plus or minus 2.2 pounds, and two actually gained weight'.

### The dangers of dieting

What mechanism does the body use to slow its metabolic rate? The most efficient would be to slow the function of the body's most metabolically active cells: those in the vital organs. The dramatic drop in metabolic rate produced by these experiments cannot be because of loss of fat, because fat is a relatively inactive part of the body. Ancel Keys proposes a mechanism that might well give any dieter pause for thought:

> It appears that the tissue loss and the changes in the metabolic rate of the liver and other organs with high metabolic rate may be of considerable importance in explaining the changes in basal metabolism during starvation and food restriction.

And he calculates that 80 per cent of the decrease in oxygen consumption in his subjects can be accounted for by a halving of the oxygen used by the liver and its associated organs.

The body needs oxygen all the time for its vital functions. The greater the body's capacity for oxygen, the fitter a person will be. A high capacity for oxygen is also the best natural preventative against diseases of the heart, lungs and blood vessels. But the consequence of dieting, Keys proposes, is dramatically to lower the body's use of oxygen. Dieting cannot in itself be a healthy activity.

Dr Apfelbaum recently reviewed the results obtained in twenty-four studies of under-nutrition made between 1903 and 1969. Men and women of widely varying weight and in different circumstances were underfed for different reasons for periods varying between three weeks and two years. The amount of energy consumed as food in these studies ranged from 1600 calories a day to 700 to 1200 (several) to zero—fasting. 'All the authors report a decrease of the basal metabolic rate as a result of diet restriction ranging from 10 to 45 per cent according to the length and stringency of the restriction.'

Professor Albert Stunkard, a leading American expert, confirms that dieting slows down the metabolic rate and frustrates the dieter. He goes on to say: 'Repeated attempts at weight reduction may lead to a progressive slowing of weight loss and to even more rapid regaining of weight.'

I have yet to read of any account of this phenomenon in any diet book. This is not surprising. The facts that the scientists have known for decades, and that have been set down in scientific journals and textbooks, make most diet books so much waste paper.

Now, in 1983, the British medical establishment is acknowledging that metabolism is dynamic. The Royal College of Physicians, referring to some of the studies summarised here, put a bomb under the diet books by saying, in its report on obesity:

> It has been known for many years that there are substantial differences in the metabolic rates of individuals at rest and also that the body is able to adapt to changes in energy intake. If volunteers are given only half their usual intake, there is an early fall in the metabolic rate of the tissues.

Dieting slows you down more than weight loss can explain because dieting slows down the processes of the most active vital organs in the body. This process can be dangerous if the diet is extreme or prolonged or unbalanced, or if the dieter is not in good health, or if the dieting is repeated over a number of years.

Millions of people, women mostly, in Great Britain, the USA and other countries go in for fad diets every year. They are damaging their health.

The more severe the diet, the more you slow down. Fasting has the most dramatic effect. 'Energy requirements decrease by 25 to 30 per cent in the course of three to four weeks of fasting,' reports Ernst Drenick, an American doctor who favours fasting as a treatment for obese patients. He goes on to say:

> Restraint should be advised in the amounts of food allowed after fasting or after the desired weight level has been attained with fasting. The adaptive lowering of the metabolic rate may quickly lead to substantial weight gains if normal, average meals are consumed during this period.

In other words, the only way not to put on the weight that has been lost by fasting is to go on a diet after the fast has ended.

### Fasting wastes muscle

Drenick subjected 137 very fat people to fasts of between one and four months. The average weight loss was 4 stone 9 pounds. The patients were well pleased. However, when 105 were followed up two years later, 96 had regained their pre-fast weight. Drenick acknowledges that during two-month fasts his subjects lost 17 pounds of muscle on average, but he does not suggest that this is why they regained weight. Instead, he says that 'regular revisits and close supervision' during the follow-up period are crucial and concludes:

> Our experiences are disappointing. [But] a sizeable number of the subjects had been on welfare for years; many of them had never been usefully employed. Therefore solid motivation over the long run might be questioned in some of these patients.

In other words, the experiment is valid, but the subjects are not up to standard—a new version of 'the operation was successful, but the patient died.' Sometimes, fasting results in death from heart failure. So does fasting modified by the administration of liquid protein, a regime made popular in America by Robert Linn's book *The Last Chance Diet*. In 1978 the American Government investigated fifty-eight cases in which this liquid protein diet had led to death from heart failure. The more extreme a diet is, the more dangerous it is.

But what happens to patients who do survive fasts? Frederick Benoit, a Californian doctor, subjected seven fat US naval personnel to a fast quick enough to tempt impatient dieters: ten days. In this time the average weight lost was just over 20 pounds. However: 'The mean weight loss from fasting was due to 64.6 per cent decrease in lean body weight and only 35.4 per cent loss in body fat.' Benoit concludes 'fasting beyond ten days may produce decreasing rates of lean tissue breakdown' but 'the wisdom of incurring such wastes in lean body tissue is open to question'.

There is something to be said for fasting. People who occasionally fast for a day or two often find the experience refreshing. But fasting is not a way to lose fat. It slows down the body's activity dramatically, to a point as close as ordinary people ever get to hibernation, and it wastes lean body tissue, including muscle, designed to be metabolically active. Fasting changes the composition of the body, so that after the fast the body works at a lower energy level than before it started, not only because weight has been lost but also because of the wasting of metabolically active tissue. Special exercises, like those used by physiotherapists to rehabilitate people whose muscles have been wasted as a result of inactivity after a surgical operation, are the only way to restore the body to its previous metabolic rate after a prolonged fast.

## Over-eating speeds you up

If dieting slows you down, and fasting slows you down even more, does it follow that over-feeding will speed up the metabolic rate? Yes, it does. Over-feeding does not make you thin, of course, but it does speed up the rate at which the body uses energy. The studies on this subject are as extensive as those on under-feeding.

In 1901, a German, R O Neumann, reported the results of an experiment upon himself, in which he over-ate for long periods. After an initial weight gain, he found that he could eat 800 calories a day above his normal intake and gain little extra weight. His conclusion was that 'someone who is healthy can take in surplus food and consume it by burning it faster.'

This experiment was repeated by Derek Miller in the 1960s, when forty-nine subjects were encouraged to eat at least 1000 calories a day above their normal intake for periods of up to eight weeks:

> There was a marked weekly adaptation to the calorie load, such that the rate of weight gain fell throughout the experiment. There was a marked individual variation, and it is quite remarkable how some individuals can eat an excess of 10,000 calories a week and show a weight loss.

After over-feeding, a person's metabolic rate when asleep and at rest speeds up, as does the energy given off as a direct result of eating. Most remarkable of all is the effect on the energy used when exercising. In one study the oxygen consumed by people who were over-eating increased by 30 per cent during walking, 25 per cent during cycling and 19 per cent during stair-climbing. Oxygen consumed during exercise is a measure of energy used. By contrast, Ernst Drenick found that after a three- to seven-week fast, oxygen consumption decreased by 21 per cent during bed rest, 32 per cent when sitting, and 40 per cent when walking.

### Different people, different speeds

Diets train the body to adapt to the circumstances of dieting, which it does by slowing down its vital functions. This adaptive behaviour is the best means of staying alive and as healthy as possible in famine. As already stated, our minds know the difference between going on a diet and famine or starvation; but our bodies do not.

Different people have different metabolic rates, for a variety of factors that help to explain why some people never get fat and other people get fat very easily. These include physical make-up, mental state, the circumstances in which people live, and their state of health; how active they are; and how fit they are. Some of these factors cannot be altered, others can be. Not only is metabolism dynamic, slowing down or speeding up according to the volume of food eaten; but it is variable at will. Dieters feel imprisoned in their bodies partly because they do not realise that they can speed up their metabolic rate. Within wide limits we can choose how much energy we want our bodies to use; it is literally a question of how lively we choose to be.

Other things being equal, a heavy person needs more energy than a light person. Someone who loses weight will use less energy and need less food simply because they are lighter. A tall person needs more energy than a short person because a larger body surface enables more heat to escape.

Because body fat is metabolically less active than fat-free tissue—muscle and the vital organs in particular—the greater the proportion of fat-free tissue in the body, the greater therefore the energy requirement. Similarly, the greater the proportion of fat in the body, the less energy required. Metabolic rates vary, and a fat person's can be higher than a thin person's because they are heavier or because, although they have a greater proportion of fat, they have a bigger body with more fat-free tissue as well. Weight for weight, though, a lean person will have a higher metabolic rate because of being lean, whereas a fat person will have a low metabolic rate because of being fat.

Men are usually heavier and taller than women with less body fat. The average woman has about 9 per cent more fat than the average man. There are three types of fat: subcutaneous, which is deposited under the skin; depot, which lies deeper, characteristically on the abdomen in men and around the hips and thighs in women; and essential fat, within the body to protect the vital organs. Women have more depot and essential body fat than men. The average man uses more energy than the average woman, not because he is a man (whatever that might mean) but because he is heavier, taller and leaner. A woman and man of the same height, weight and body composition will have the same energy requirements.

### Energy breeds energy

From adulthood onwards, energy requirements decline by about 5 per cent a decade. It follows that the average 60-year-old requires about 20 per cent less food than the average 20-year-old. The World Health Organisation's recommended figures for daily energy intake from food are:

| age | men (11 st) calories | women (8 st 8 lb) calories |
|---|---|---|
| 16–19 | 3600 | 2400 |
| 20–29 | 3200 | 2300 |
| 30–39 | 3100 | 2200 |
| 40–49 | 3000 | 2200 |
| 50–59 | 2800 | 2000 |
| 60–69 | 2500 | 1800 |
| 70 + | 2200 | 1600 |

It is true that maximum oxygen capacity, a measure of physical energy requirement, declines slowly as a function of age, at a rate of about 2 per cent a decade. But these figures mostly reflect the fact that what exercise young people in the West do take declines almost to zero in middle age. People who remain active into old age continue to need, and to use, high amounts of energy. Elderly Swiss farmers of both sexes have been observed to have an energy requirement as high as 4000 to 5000 calories a day.

The sedentary man or woman who becomes less active but eats more in middle age is in trouble. Having said that the significance of physical activity in weight gain in middle age has up to now been under-emphasised, the Royal College of Physicians report on obesity states:

Increasing inactivity in middle age forms the basis for the decline in muscle mass and lean body mass as people grow older. The replacement of lean tissue by fat with ageing compounds the problem of energy balance since the basal need for energy falls with the reduction in metabolically active lean tissue; this will lead to a further drop in the basal metabolic rate and a tendency to gain body fat.

As a rule, adolescents require more energy than adults, for their growth as well as their activity. Pregnant women need about 300 extra calories a day; lactating women, about 500 extra calories a day.

A very small number of people suffer from a disorder of their metabolic function and become grossly obese despite eating normal amounts of food. These people do indeed have 'something wrong with their glands'. A number of the patients hospitalised in obesity wards are dangerously overweight for such reasons and, simply because they are available to doctors, have been much studied. Without treatment of the underlying cause of their obesity, not much can be done for them long-term by diet regimes.

Recent work done by Dr Michael Stock and Nancy Rothwell in London indicates that a special type of body fat, brown fat, present in small but variable quantities at various sites in the body, is very active metabolically. Most of the work done on brown fat has been carried out on rats, and it is not yet known whether we can increase our brown fat stores and so burn energy faster.

To say that someone has a high metabolic rate is to say, in scientific terms, that they use a lot of energy. An energetic person will tend to use those parts of the body that are themselves metabolically active and will therefore need and use more energy at rest and when active. One effect of diet books is to discourage us from taking account of what, given reflection and self-awareness, we already know: energy breeds energy.

Mental and emotional states, and physical health, also affect the speed at which our bodies work. Being 'high' or 'low' is not just a mental state; it reflects high or low biochemical states. Elation and fever are two examples of high states, one good, one bad; both require and use more energy. Depression literally depresses the body's energy. A person in a low mental state may gain fat not because they eat more food but because the food they are eating, normally the right amount, is too much in a depressed state. The depressed person who worries about weight but is unaware that depression affects the rate at which the body uses energy is in a vicious circle. Lacking guidance, they are liable to eat a normal amount of food, gain fat, and so become more depressed. If a pattern is established, the result may be self-destructive behaviour, such as eating abnormally large quantities of food.

People in industrialised societies have lost touch with their bodies. But animals that become out of sorts or physically depressed, for whatever reason, spend a lot of time resting and sleeping. So do people in tribal societies. The body has its own energy resources. Pressing food on someone who is ill is usually completely the wrong thing to do; the body's energy needs to be directed to the source of the illness, not to digestion.

### Lean people use most energy

The common experience of one particularly strong emotion, the state of 'being in love', is that the lover refuses food when he or she is secretly pining after the loved one. If Romeo and Juliet wanted to lose weight in the first part of their play, they were in luck. But if love has the lineaments of gratified desire and is altogether active, not passive, then the Tom Jones syndrome applies, and the lover is liable to eat with the appetite of the furnace of a steam locomotive.

This account of the physical, mental and emotional circumstances that determine and change metabolic rate, and also of the amount of energy the body needs and uses, is really nothing more than common sense. Dieting depresses the human organism. And the mental depression that follows dieting is caused by this physical depression. Dieting slows down the spirit as well as the body. Christian evangelists preach the mortification of the flesh as the only means to achieve grace. Diet books substitute health for faith but otherwise use the same techniques. And the promises made by diet books are illusions.

The more you weigh, and the more lean body tissue you have, the higher your metabolic rate will tend to be at all times—when asleep, when resting and when active.

Most tables of energy requirements, for example those published by the World Health Organisation, give body weight as the only variable factor affecting basal metabolic rate (that is, the speed at which the body works at complete rest, with no food to digest). This is fair enough for most populations in the world. But for Western people, who tend to get fat, the tables, which are the source for the statements made in diet books about the amount of energy from food (calories) we require, are misleading. They imply that a light person has a low metabolic rate just because they are light and that a heavy person has a high metabolic rate just because they are heavy: and this is not accurate.

The lowest metabolic rate is that of someone who, as well as being light, is also fat; the highest metabolic rate is that of someone who, as well as being heavy, is also lean. It follows therefore that a light, lean person may have the same metabolic rate as a heavy, fat person. Laboratory experiments carried out by Professor John Durnin show that it is possible for a lean person weighing 8 stone to need and use the same amount of energy as a fat person weighing 11 stone.

The calories per day required at rest by people of different weights and body composition shown here are recalculated from the tables originally devised by Professor Durnin. The figures are of course approximations:

| *Men* | *Women* | *7st 12lb* | *9st 6lb* | *11st* | *12st 8lb* | *14st 2lb* |
|---|---|---|---|---|---|---|
| Lean | | 1450 | 1650 | 1850 | 2050 | 2250 |
| Average | Lean | 1300 | 1500 | 1700 | 1900 | 2100 |
| Fat | Average | 1150 | 1350 | 1550 | 1750 | 1950 |
| Obese | Fat | 1000 | 1200 | 1400 | 1600 | 1800 |
| | Obese | 850 | 1050 | 1250 | 1450 | 1650 |

The figures for men and women are different not only because of the difference in weights but also because the terms 'lean' and 'fat' are relative: a lean man has about 10 per cent body fat, taking subcutaneous, depot and essential fat together, whereas a lean woman has about 20 per cent body fat. Therefore, a lean woman of the same body weight as a lean man is less metabolically active.

Thus the average man of 11 stone already referred to uses about 1700 calories at rest; the average woman of 8 stone 8 pounds around 1250 calories.

This is one reason why the middle-aged sedentary woman can indeed 'eat like a bird' and yet continue to gain weight and fat, whereas the active man can 'eat like a horse' and yet stay lean. A very active, lean young man of 14 stone 2 pounds requires as much and more energy for his activity as for his basic vital functions and might need 5000 calories a day, or even more. By contrast an inactive, small woman in her fifties with little lean tissue could gain fat on no more than 1200 calories a day—even less, in the case of women who have wasted away their lean tissue by continual diet regimes. With the almost universal use of cars as a means of transport, and diets as a means of slimming, in the West in the last thirty years, millions of Western women are in energy balance at artificially low levels, so low as to damage their health.

### Fat regained

If a fat woman of, say, 11 stone could, by dieting, reduce to 8 stone, and if the diet worked according to her dream, so that all the weight lost was fat, then she could eat as much food at the lean weight of 8 stone as she previously did at the fat weight of 11 stone. But this dream is a fantasy which—as most dieters know—is liable to become a waking nightmare.

When a diet has ended, the body will replace the glycogen and water it has lost: these are essential to its vital functions. How much weight these represent depends of course on how much they have been depleted by the diet. As a rule any diet that has led to a loss of 10 to 15 pounds in the first week or two will also lead to a gain of 10 to 15 pounds in a week or two after the diet has ended. Dieters should know that the reason is because such diets drain glycogen and water; the gaining of weight is not their fault, and doctors and books blaming them are in effect perpetrating a cruel hoax.

It is of course true that any diet will result in a loss of fat. But the metabolically active tissue lost on a diet has the effect of artificially depressing the body's energy needs. To take just one example, a woman who loses 20 pounds on a diet might previously have needed 2000 calories a day from food but no more than 1500 afterwards. If she—and any other dieter—is prepared to follow the diet with an indefinite modified diet, then she could keep off the fat lost on the diet, at the expense of becoming rather weak and perpetually depriving herself of food a healthy baby needs.

It is also true that if, after a diet, a lighter person becomes considerably more active, and so uses more energy in exercise and also builds up metabolically active lean tissue, then they can not only keep off the fat lost, but also eat more and at the same time become leaner. The happy people who become active after a diet, because they like the look of themselves at a lighter weight, become slim not because they dieted but because they followed their diet with exercise. The only people I know who have kept much weight off in the long term after a diet has ended are those who started to exercise regularly during or after the diet.

The fact is that most people regain the weight lost on a diet. In her book *Fat is a Feminist Issue*, Susie Orbach claims that in the long term 95 per cent of all dieters regain all the weight lost on diet regimes. This figure, which is quite often cited, is open to doubt. But it is safe to say that the eventual result of dieting is as likely to be a net weight gain as a net weight loss. The Royal College of Physicians report on obesity states:

Maintenance of weight loss beyond one year was less satisfactory and all longer-term studies have found that weight increases again in the majority of patients. In the most complete study, 154 of the 190 patients who had been treated one to five years previously were found for questioning. Twenty-five (16 per cent) had maintained a weight loss of over 40 pounds and 27 (17 per cent) were heavier than at the start of the study.

Very few people indeed eat sparingly immediately after a diet has ended. Almost invariably they respond to the body's cravings by eating at least as much as they ate before the diet started. This is not because of habit, nor, however much the dieters may blame themselves, because of greed, stupidity or thoughtlessness. The body needs energy to regenerate and responds to the first days after a diet has ended with signals of extreme hunger.

And woe to the sedentary dieter. Once the glycogen and water has been replaced, the body of the sedentary person, being used to fat, will tend to regain fat and will rebuild muscle less, simply because muscle is used less by an inactive person. For a sedentary person the result of a diet, once weight has been regained after it has ended, is to alter the composition of the body. The proportion of lean tissue in the body decreases; the proportion of fatty tissue increases. Muscle is lost; fat is gained. This is one of the reasons why dieting makes you fat.

Nobody ever became fat in a concentration camp. But the survivors of concentration camps who resumed sedentary lives did tend to become fat. Prison camp diets devastate muscle. The people who survived Hitler's death camps frequently became very flabby after the war; not necessarily heavy, but fat.

The consequences of a single diet regime, even if severe and prolonged, for a sedentary person, need not be damaging. The change in composition of the body after one diet is unlikely to be dramatic. All the same, Dr Garrow's comment on Benedict's 60-day and Keys' 24-week experiments is a warning to any optimist willing to trust to willpower:

It is interesting that the volunteers for the semi-starvation experiments of Benedict et al (1919) and Keys et al (1950) tended to over-eat and become obese after the termination of the experiment.

In both cases 'semi-starvation' consisted of regimes of 1500 calories a day. After his experiment was over, Keys put his subjects on a gradual re-feeding programme, of the kind all diet books recommend as sensible. The men remained ravenous. After the re-feeding programme ended and the men could eat as much as they liked, some became ill from over-eating; they averaged a consumption of 5000 calories a day; and regained their pre-diet weights without regaining all their muscle tissue. They ended up fatter than they started.

### Energy lost

For a sedentary person a lifetime spent between diets is not only self-defeating but also dangerous. Every diet trains the body to adapt to dieting, which it does by slowing itself down, losing some lean tissue and not replacing all of it. Every diet alters the composition of the body cumulatively.

Dieting makes you fat because of this cumulative change in the composition of the body. A second reason why dieting makes you fat is that fat is lighter than muscle. The net result of a diet, for a sedentary person, may be a loss of weight. But the body of such a dieter may nevertheless contain a greater proportion of fat. Certainly any sedentary dieter who regains the weight lost after a diet is bound to be fatter than when they started, simply because they will have replaced heavier muscle with lighter and bulkier fat.

A third reason why dieting makes you fat is because fat is less metabolically active than muscle. The greater the proportion of fat in the body, the lower the metabolic rate of that body and, therefore, the less energy required from food. Paradoxically, this process is a sign that the body is functioning efficiently; the most self-protective reaction the body can have to a diet regime, which it construes as a state of famine, is to adapt the better to survive the next famine. This it does best by requiring less food and by storing more fat.

For a sedentary person, the one sure way to slow the body

down and so create the conditions for getting fat is to go on a diet. Every diet trains the body to become less energetic, to require less energy from food, and to use less energy from oxygen with which to burn food. The habitual dieter is on a downward spiral which remorselessly reduces their vitality.

This is why dieting makes you fat.

But why does up to half the population of Great Britain, the USA and other industrialised societies steadily gain weight and fat throughout life? Why do we get fat in the first place?

# CHAPTER THREE

# Sugar Makes You Hungry

The aspects of things that are most important for us are hidden because of their simplicity and familiarity. One is unable to notice something—because it is always before one's eyes. We fail to be struck by what, once seen, is most striking and most powerful.
LUDWIG WITTGENSTEIN
*Philosophical Investigations*

Breathing at my side, that heavy animal,
That heavy bear that sleeps with me,
Howls in his sleep for a world of sugar,
A sweetness intimate as the water's clasp.
DELMORE SCHWARTZ
*The Heavy Bear That Goes With Me*

## Why do we get fat?

For every dieter there's another man or woman who doesn't diet but who gets fat all the same. Nobody wants to be fat. Yet most people over the age of 30 in Great Britain, the USA and other countries will acknowledge that they'd like to lose some weight (meaning, fat, of course). That is why diet books have such massive sales.

Every year scores of millions of people in the West go on diets; which don't work. Scores of millions more people get fat without going on diets. People in industrialised societies have tended to get fatter and fatter during this century. The trend is continuing.

A year never goes by without a representative body of scientists or doctors in the USA or Great Britain stating, again, that obesity is a massive public health problem. An American team of experts with a sense of humour recently worked out that the US adult population was carrying a total of 2297 million pounds of excess fat which, if converted into energy, would be enough to supply the annual residential electricity demands of Boston, Chicago, San Francisco and Washington.

It was not always so. Dieting is almost entirely a twentieth-century phenomenon. One hundred years ago and more, few people dieted—because they didn't need to. Few, other than the rich (whose faces are commemorated in paintings) and dandies like Byron, tended to get fat. And dieting is almost entirely a Western phenomenon. There still are very many millions of people in the world living away from Western influence—hunter-gatherers, pastoralists, farmers, peasants and people in remote countries—who may eat well, live to a ripe old age, but do not tend to gain weight and get fat as they get older. In the Third World it is only when people move from the countryside to the towns, or when they start to eat Western-influenced food, that they put on fat. It is the rich (whose pictures we see in the papers and on television) who most commonly get fat.

Diet books and most obesity textbooks assume that we get fat because we are eating more and more. Some people of course do get fat because they eat great quantities of food. But greed is not the usual reason. Overall, people in the West are eating less and less while becoming fatter and fatter. What, then, can be the cause of our overweight?

The massive difference between the food we in the West eat and the food eaten by everyone until this century is a difference primarily not of quantity, but of quality. Measured in the conventional way, we eat about the same amount of protein as do people in the Third World who live in settled societies; rather less carbohydrate; and a great deal more fat. The most impressive difference, though, is between whole food and processed food. In particular, all studies made of the differences between the foods eaten in Western and non-Western societies show that people in the West eat great amounts of processed carbohydrate, refined sugar especially; whereas people who live away from Western influence, including people in Western countries which are little influenced by industrialisation, eat great amounts of whole carbohydrate, starch especially. And people in the West get fat, whereas, as a rule, non-Western people do not.

It makes sense to discover whether the connection between processed carbohydrates, refined sugar in particular, and fatness is causal or merely coincidental.

## The rise of the sweet tooth

Until recently sugar was a luxury. In 1300 AD a pound of refined sugar cost a year's pay; sugar then was a chic item on the tables of the cosmopolitan rich, much as caviare is today. In 1700, Great Britain was importing 20 million pounds of refined sugar a year; in 1800, 160 million pounds. Sugar was of course the main non-human commodity of the slave trade, which helped to make Great Britain the richest and most powerful nation in the world. By 1850 consumption of refined sugar had risen to about 20 pounds a person a year. The tax on sugar helped to pay for the Crimean War. In 1874 Gladstone removed the tax on sugar, and consumption rose steeply, so that in 1900 every man, woman and child in Great Britain was eating an average of 72 pounds of refined sugar a year, and expenditure on sugar matched that on bread. The British sweet tooth was bred a century ago, and it was then that sweet foods became popular in shops and at home.

Consumption of refined sugar continued to rise during this century, except during the two world wars. By the mid-1950s, with sweets and confectionery off the ration again, the British were eating more refined sugar than ever before. For the last 30 years the volume of sugar manufactured in and imported to Great Britain has been of the order of 2,500,000 tons a year, or around 100 pounds for every man, woman and child.

The average consumption of refined sugar in Great Britain is therefore about 5 ounces a day, a head. The energy content of 5 ounces of sugar is about 550 calories; which is to say, 18 to 24 per cent of the energy requirement from food for the average, lightly active adult.

The world average consumption of refined sugar is now about one-third of the British figure. The overall African figure is about one-fifth, but is rising. The overall Asian figure is about one-eighth, but is also rising. Wherever Coca-Cola signs can be found, more and more refined sugar is being eaten.

There was a time when the British ate more refined sugar than any other nation; that time has now passed. People in Mediterranean countries still eat less of it; but 100 pounds a year is, as a round figure, accurate for North America, Europe and other developed countries.

In Great Britain roughly half of all refined sugar eaten is contained within manufactured food, and of this well over half is in chocolate, confectionery, cakes, biscuits and soft drinks. Chocolate is over half sugar; sweets are almost all sugar; a Mars Bar, the most popular British confectionery line, is 65.8 per cent sugar; biscuits vary between 10 and 45 per cent sugar; soft drinks such as Coca-Cola are about 90 per cent water and 10 per cent sugar.

Some people eat less, some more, than the average of 100 pounds a year or 5 ounces a day of refined sugar. Adolescents and young men and women without the means or inclination to prepare or buy their own meals, who snack a lot, may eat 200 pounds a year, or even more; a figure approaching, or even greater than, half their energy requirement from food. It is believed that in the USA, Canada and Britain some teenage boys consume up to 400 pounds of refined sugar a year.

To someone without a sweet tooth the figure of 100 pounds a year, which includes only processed, 'refined', sugar but not natural sugars in fruit and some vegetables, may seem remarkably high. But refined sugar is used very extensively by food manufacturers.

Some foods regarded as healthy, or at least not thought of as sweet, contain a lot of refined sugar, as the table 'Sugar in Food' on pages 108–11 shows. Sweet pickle is about one-third refined sugar. Canned fruits with syrup total about one-quarter refined sugar; as do tomato ketchup and packet muesli. Flavoured and fruit yogurt is between 13 and 18 per cent refined sugar; baked beans are over 5 per cent. Varying amounts of refined sugar are added to soups; diluted with an equal amount of water, condensed cream of tomato soup is 5.6 per cent refined sugar. Anyone who wants to avoid eating refined sugar has to be alert.

In Great Britain and the USA there is now a trend towards eating less refined sugar at home, but more away from home. In Great Britain, Mars Bars were first manufactured in 1932. Fifty years later, 700 million were sold. Between 1932 and 1982 the amount of confectionery eaten per head went up from 5½ ounces to 8 ounces a week—the extra 2½ ounces being the weight of one Mars Bar, which contains a total of 320 calories of energy.

Refined sugar is inert. It contains no vitamins and only the faintest traces of some other nutrients. In this, alone of all the foods we consume in any quantity, it is comparable only with alcoholic spirits. It supplies dead, or empty, energy. And the very last food that is suitable for a basically sedentary population is food that supplies nothing but energy. Almost all brown sugar also contains no nourishment. Sugar sold as 'raw cane' sugar has some nourishment remaining.

We have been taught that the principal requirement of the human body is for quantity: readily measurable energy. This is wrong. Our principal requirement is for quality: hard-to-measure nourishment. And refined sugar, alone among all the substances we eat, has been processed so thoroughly that it has no nutritive value.

The advertisements of manufacturers of products sweetened by refined sugar foster the notion that the energy in food is used mostly for activity. This is not true. As stated above, the lightly active person, who compensates for a sedentary job by walking, gardening, golf or other regular weekend and holiday activity, uses only one-third of the energy supplied by food for activity; the other two-thirds go to fuel the body's basic functions, and digestion. And our body needs nourishment from vitamins, minerals and other nutrients, not merely energy.

Throughout this century people in the West have become less active. The car has replaced walking. Machines do housework and gardening. Much work on the farm, in factories and on building sites has been automated. People even buy electric carving knives. And yet, at the same time, more and more of the food we eat has nourishment processed out of it; and, in the case of refined sugar, has no nourishment in it at all.

### Low energy, poor nourishment

I asked Arvid Wretlind about the consequences of this. Professor Wretlind, a world authority on vitamins, works for the National Institute of Public Health in Stockholm and has made a special study of the nutrition problems of people who consume small amounts of food.

He pointed out that the nutritional requirements of men and women from vitamins and minerals correspond to pre-twentieth-century energy levels. Until this century, people obtained nourishment from food supplying 2500 to 3000 calories a day or more, because their regular physical activity required a calorie intake at that level. Wretlind explains:

> The lower the physical activity the higher will be the content of the essential nutrients required per calorie in order to obtain the desired, optimal, nutritional level. A diet which is adequate for a man with a calorie requirement of 3000 calories a day cannot simply be assumed to cover the desirable nutritional supply for a low calorie consumer—for example, a woman with a calorie requirement of less than 2000 calories a day.

That is to say, people with a low energy intake need to eat especially nutritious food to make sure of getting enough vitamins and minerals. Studies show that varying groups of people with a low energy intake receive insufficient nutrients, for example vitamin A (carotene), riboflavin (vitamin B2), vitamin C (ascorbic acid), calcium and iron. Wretlind's conclusion is that:

> The low caloric group, such as schoolgirls, office girls, women, and old-age pensioners do not receive a supply of nutrients corresponding to that considered desirable for good nutritional conditions.

Here he is describing healthy people of normal habits; or, at least, superficially healthy people, for he goes on to say that in Sweden, and in countries like Sweden, 'a number of disturbances occur in the state of health and well-being which are either wholly or partially due to the unsuitable composition of the diet or to defective dietary habits.'

When you think about it, this view is common sense. Take an average-size woman who, before this century, would have been in energy balance eating nourishing food with an energy value of say 2500 calories. The equivalent woman of the same height now, who has an office job, will be in energy balance at about 2000 calories a day, even if she takes a little exercise. Already, therefore, she can only be getting 80 per cent of the nourishment her body needs.

Now assume that she is eating an average amount of refined sugar, supplying 550 calories daily. It follows that she is consuming 1450 nourishing calories daily, even on the assumption that all the rest of the food she is eating is nourishing. Call it 1500 to round the figures. She is therefore getting only 60 per cent of the nourishment her body needs. I would describe that as a state of mild but permanent malnutrition, suffered not only by women and office girls but by men with office jobs too.

Refined sugar is not, though, the only food we eat that is short of nourishment. The process of manufacture removes nutrients from staple foods—white flour, white bread, white rice for example. Beri-beri, a deficiency disease caused by severe lack of thiamine (vitamin B1), became rampant in the late nineteenth century in the Dutch East Indies not among the very poor, who continued to eat whole, brown rice, but among those who could afford the new polished, white rice made by machines imported from Europe.

The ideal food commodity is cheap, easily transported, does not rot, preserves other foods and is highly palatable. Food is processed not in order to be more nourishing but in order to become a better commodity; to make more money. It is not by chance that Great Britain became the richest nation on earth partly by means of the profits from sugar. All manufactured foods lose nourishment. Any food advertised as having vitamins and minerals added is usually food which has lost vitamins and minerals in the process of manufacture.

## We get fat in order to stay healthy

Yet more nutrients are lost in the process of preparation and cooking. Generally speaking, the more sophisticated these processes, the more nourishment is lost. (The original meaning of 'sophistication' was 'adulteration'. Brewers in previous centuries who 'sophisticated' their beer with sugar were fined or beaten.) Japanese food, celebrated as among the most healthy in the world, is undercooked. We in the West discard much of the most nutritious parts of food—skin, peel, pith from fruit and vegetables, blood and guts from meat. Then we overcook what we choose to eat, with the result that the water-soluble vitamins B and C go down the drain and many other nutrients go up in smoke.

There is no way of estimating how many nutrients are lost by manufacture and in cooking. Nor does anyone know what is the precise effect on the body of contamination of the air and of food by pesticides, chemicals and drugs. We are aware that nuclear fall-out has hidden long-term effects. But what effects do hormones injected into animals to make them more profitable commodities eventually have on the body of the consumer? We just don't know. What we do know is that one use the body makes of vitamins is to resist infection and also to resist poisoning from its own toxins; and these vitamins can be marshalled by the body as a means of resisting outside contamination. It follows, therefore, that the more contamination there is in the air and in food, the more the body's resources will be depleted, even exhausted.

None of this takes dieting into account. What happens if someone who is normally getting about half the nourishment their body needs goes on a diet regime supplying, say, 1000 calories a day? Unless the diet eliminates all refined sugar, all other processed food, and the dieter ensures that all food eaten is fresh, lightly cooked and nourishing, the body will suffer a sharp shock and will be jerked from a state of mild malnutrition to one of acute, even severe malnutrition.

From the body's point of view, the significant change is not the drop of energy intake; we have always been able to adjust to scarcity and famine, which frustrate the dieter. The starvation that the weight-conscious dieter, man or woman, suffers is not of energy but of nourishment.

Here is another reason for the raging appetite the dieter develops after the diet has ended. This compulsion for food can so baffle and overwhelm the dieter that it becomes a genuinely frightening experience. The healthy body can adjust to a period of emergency, which in effect is what a diet is; but, once the emergency is over, the body's imperative demand is for the nourishment that succours it.

We in the West become overweight against our will, and without being greedy consume more energy from food than our bodies require, because this is the only way our bodies can get enough nourishment. We become overweight as a means of staying healthy. The overweight person who is well known for always being in a good mood is someone who has come to terms with being overweight—or, frankly, fat. Their well-being springs not from being overweight, but from getting enough nourishment from food. Such people tend to level out at a weight and percentage of fat well above the 'desirable' level, once the size of their body corresponds to a volume of food containing adequate nourishment.

When sedentary or even moderately active people eat sugar

and other refined foods the only way they can get enough nourishment is to consume more energy than their bodies require. A vigorously active person can burn off these extra, empty calories; a less active person cannot. A sedentary person has the choice of eventually becoming overweight and then fat; or of being under-nourished and suffering from malaise and then illness. This is why healthy dieters find slimming such a frustrating process. The body's defence and protection mechanisms overpower the mind's desire for the body to become an 'ideal' weight or shape. Ironically, though, in time becoming fat itself is liable to bring illness with it.

'Sugar is an unnecessary source of energy in a community with such a widespread problem of overweight,' stated the Royal College of Physicians in their 1983 report on obesity. The report went on to confirm that sugar is not only without value but also deprives us of the vitamins and minerals we would otherwise eat in healthy food: 'A halving of the average sugar consumption per head of the population would increase the nutrient/energy density of the diet. This would ensure that mineral and vitamin requirements were more likely to be met.'

Members of the Royal College working party have confirmed to me that the report recommended a halving of sugar consumption, rather than cutting it out altogether, for practical, not medical, reasons. The Royal College has a responsibility to produce reports acceptable to the public and also, it is to be hoped, to the Department of Health. There is a limit beyond which no representative body is likely to go in advocating radical proposals. Nevertheless, the Royal College does make it quite clear that refined sugar is unnecessary and deprives us of vitamins and minerals we need.

### Deficiency states

What are the consequences of eating refined sugar? Deficiency diseases are caused by lack of nutrients: by malnutrition, not only by under-nutrition. Some diseases caused by lack of vitamins became epidemic in Western countries in the past among populations whose food was very unbalanced, usually because of unnatural living habits, as among the newly industrialised poor or on board ship. Other such diseases are regarded as exotic. Scurvy (caused by lack of vitamin C, or ascorbic acid) was commonplace among British sailors until lemons and limes were identified as a preventative. Rickets (lack of vitamin D) was commonplace among children of the urban poor in Britain until 50 years ago. Xerophthalmia (lack of vitamin A) causes blindness in hundreds of thousands of children in the Third World. Beri-beri (lack of thiamine, or vitamin B1) still occurs particularly among peoples in Asia whose staple cereal is processed, white rice. Pellagra (lack of niacin, or vitamin B3) was rampant in the southern states of America among people whose staple diet was corn.

As more vitamins are identified, more diseases caused by deficiency of these nutrients are also identified, diseases which do not have names as resonant as 'scurvy' or 'beri-beri'. Other vitamins classified as within the B group, are pyridoxine (B6), pantothenic acid, biotin, folic acid, B12, choline, inositol and para-amino-benzoic acid (PABA). More vitamins are being identified and given more mind-numbing names.

If the food we ate were nutritious and well-balanced, and if we were active enough to need enough food to supply enough nourishment, then we would have no need to become aware of vitamins. Casimir Funk, who identified polished rice as the cause of beri-beri in London in 1912 and who coined the name 'vitamin' (meaning VITal AMINo acid) was opposed to the system whereby food manufacturers extract and discard nutrients from food, which they defend by adding synthetic versions of those vitamins so far identified as having been destroyed. He said:

Vitamins are not any magical possessions. They exist in milk because the mother or the cow assemble them from the food she has eaten. What would be the use of preparing all our foods artificially as long as nature is producing her own foods in sufficient abundance?

Half a century later the USA and the West still produce food in abundance. In November 1982 the total amount of butter, cheese and skimmed milk cached in America was 2399 million pounds; but this dairy produce will not be sold anywhere unless the price is right for the American farmer. Agriculture and food manufacture are very big multinational business. So is the manufacture of vitamin pills.

In their clinical form, caused by gross malnutrition, deficiency diseases are easy to diagnose. But deficiency states also take mild forms that are not readily identifiable. Dr Donald McLaren, in his standard textbook *Nutrition and Its Disorders*, says:

> Malnutrition means disordered nutrition. Nutrition becomes disordered as a result of any deviation from normal. While gross deviations give rise to frank clinical signs and symptoms and definite biochemical abnormalities it is virtually impossible to draw a line between the 'normal' and the 'abnormal'.

McLaren and other doctors reckon that large numbers of people in Western countries are short of certain vitamins and minerals. Surveys have shown that 36 per cent of American women and 26 per cent of Swiss women are short of pyridoxine (B6). McLaren himself believes that deficiency of folic acid is the most common. A nutritionist at the University of Surrey has told me that 60 per cent of a group of people she studied were short of the recommended intake of folic acid (B complex), and 30 to 40 per cent were short of pyridoxine. And she was studying young athletes who were eating a lot of food—much of it, though, junk food. American surveys show that a quarter of the population is deficient in zinc, calcium and magnesium.

A problem with these findings is nobody really knows what the right level of vitamin and mineral intake should be, particularly in the case of vitamins which have always been eaten in fresh food but which have only recently been isolated by scientists. The recommended intakes are rules of thumb. Moreover, they vary from country to country: in the USA the official recommendation is, for example, 60 mg of vitamin C a day; in day; in Great Britain, the figure is 30 mg a day. Critics of the British figure say that it is so low as only to prevent signs of manifest scurvy.

Books are written about individual vitamins. Take one, folic acid. If it is deficient, red blood cells become large, abnormally shaped and short-lived. The result is a form of anaemia, common among women, especially if they need extra nourishment, when menstruating or pregnant. The symptoms are not obvious or sudden and are not likely to be diagnosed as vitamin deficiency. The victim eventually becomes weak, tired, irritable, and sometimes forgetful and sleepy.

And the result? The woman short of folic acid wonders if she could do with a drug, a pep pill or even a bar of chocolate. It is revealing to watch television commercials put out in the afternoon, for mothers and housewives: advertisements for confectionery alternate with advertisements for over-the-counter drugs. The advertisers know what they are doing.

## Malnutrition in the West

Doctors acknowledge that a high percentage of their patients complain of unspecific ailments. These include stomach discomfort, loss of appetite, anxiety, backache, constant tiredness, muscle weakness, jumpiness, digestive trouble, headaches, inability to sleep, difficulty in paying attention, nervousness—or 'general malaise', as millions of doctors' certificates put it. Any of these conditions is depressing; all zest for life and sense of well-being is lost. All these complaints can be a result of malnutrition. Certainly, most people in the West do not eat enough nutritious food, and some large groups of people, including students, office workers, old people and dieters, are especially at risk.

Scurvy is generally assumed to have vanished before the end of the sailing ship era. Not at all. In its mild form, scurvy leads to bleeding, notably from the gums, and to fragile bones. Later the joints and muscles bleed, and teeth fall out. McLaren:

Elderly bachelors and widowers who cook for themselves or eat in restaurants are particularly prone. Women, even when living alone, are better able to fend for themselves, and fruit and vegetables have a more prominent place in their diet.

Vitamin C is used by the body to resist attacks from poisonous substances, such as lead, cadmium, and carbon monoxide from exhaust fumes and from tobacco smoke. Smoking is estimated to lower the vitamin C content of the blood by 25 to 50 per cent. Alcohol has a similar effect. So have some drugs—aspirin, for example. The more we are exposed to drugs, poisons and contamination in the air and in our food, the more we need vitamins.

Moreover, foods lose nourishment by being grown in poor soil; by being picked before they are ripe; and by being preserved, dyed or waxed. And no scientist can say what effect the cocktails of chemicals we all eat and breathe is having on our health.

It is not necessary to become a campaigner or a crank to transform the quality of the food we eat. Salt is an additive which, because it is inert, does us no good. Any inert substance leaches nourishment, including vitamins, from the alimentary tract. The same is true of refined sugar. But sugar, once used as an additive as sparingly as salt, is now a staple of our diet. We eat far more sugar than any other single substance. It is incorporated into every kind of manufactured food. And we can do something about refined sugar. We can stop eating it.

In the financial year 1981 the British Sugar Corporation turned over £488,200,000, and made a profit of £51,035,000. Projected profits for 1982 were £64 million. In 1981 the British government sold its 24 per cent share in what is now British Sugar for £44 million—but it has not yet mounted a campaign against excessive consumption of refined sugar.

Sugar causes states of malnutrition in sedentary people because it replaces nourishing food and because it is a parasitical agent, draining nourishment from the body. But that is not all.

Thiamine (vitamin B1) assists the metabolic functioning of

body cells, notably nervous tissue, and the digestion. Niacin (vitamin B3) dilates the blood vessels and reduces the level of cholesterol in the blood. Both are soluble in water and so are lost in cooking, especially over-cooking. Both are attacked by sugar, and by alcohol, which in this respect has the same biochemical effects as sugar.

'Beri-Beri Menace Down at the Local' ran a headline in the *Star* on 27 October 1982. The Scottish Medical Journal had identified beri-beri among heavy beer drinkers. 'Previously it had been found only among beer drinkers in Australia, Germany and the Bantu tribal areas of South Africa,' said the report, adding that doctors wanted thiamine to be added to beer.

> But last night Angus Meldrum, marketing director of Tennant Caledonian brewers, hit out. He said 'We've no intention of doctoring our beer to meet the drinking habits of Bantu tribesmen. Thiamine this week—what next? Scots don't drink jungle juice.

That is what happens when a particular vitamin deficiency disease bears an exotic name. In North America and Europe beri-beri is not uncommon in the chronic alcoholic patient, according to McLaren. And of pellagra, caused by niacin (vitamin B3) deficiency; he writes that 'alcoholism may constitute an obstinate barrier to eradication'.

In its clinical form, diagnosed by the Scottish doctors, beri-beri, or polyneuritis, causes tingling in the hands and feet, severe mental confusion and, eventually, heart failure. In a mild form it causes fatigue, weight loss and loss of appetite, constant lassitude and sleeplessness, faulty memory and emotional instability. Serenity and zest are lost. Mild pellagra is often confused with schizophrenic states. Other symptoms, including dizziness and faintness, are similar to mild beri-beri.

There is good reason to believe that mild forms of deficiency diseases (also known as 'sub-clinical deficiency diseases' or 'deficiency states') are so common in the West that both the sufferers and their doctors fail to see what the problem is. If I feel ill but nobody else does, I know I have a problem. But if a lot of people feel fairly ill a lot of the time everybody starts to assume that the condition is normal.


## The junk food syndrome

Given that the effect of refined sugar, like alcohol, is to attack vitamin B in the body, it follows that one section of the population especially at risk is young people who consume a great deal of 'junk food' with a heavy refined sugar content.

This was what Dr Derrick Lonsdale and Dr Raymond Shamberger of Cleveland, Ohio, found in 1980. They noted symptoms of thiamine (vitamin B1) deficiency so severe as to be identifiable as an early state of beri-beri, and their report in the *American Journal of Clinical Nutrition* made clear that the problem of these young people was that they were eating junk food, or 'empty' or 'naked' calories—energy with no nourishment.

The doctors noted severe restlessness during sleep, frightening dreams, and recurrent fever diagnosed as infections by the family doctor. One syndrome was as follows:

The patient was described as unusually irritable, sensitive to criticism, becoming angered easily and showing poor impulse control, as in the case of a 17 year old male who had put his fist through a plate glass window.

Lonsdale and Shamberger even translated a Japanese treatise on beri-beri into English, finding that many aspects of the disease, 'forgotten in societies where it is believed that the condition is extinct', imitate other well-recognised diseases, because beri-beri affects all the organs and deranges energy metabolism. Their patients were treated with thiamine supplements, and all improved.

Some patients lost their craving for sweet tasting foods and beverages, although in some cases the process was extremely difficult and the temptation to succumb quite similar to that seen in people who express a wish to stop smoking.

The common assumption that diseases of malnutrition only occur among poor people eating simple food is wrong. Just as beri-beri in the East was and is caused by eating white rice, rather than the cheaper brown rice, and little other nutritious food, so Lonsdale and Shamberger's patients were all-American kids eating all-American food.

Many of them had no breakfast at all; most had school lunch and an evening meal was provided at home. In most cases it was between-meals snacking of so-called junk foods, and above all the consumption of a variety of sweet beverages that provided the empty calories.

Almost as an aside, the doctors then make a fascinating deduction from experiments with animals: 'Anorexia may be regarded as a protective device and this is well seen in experimental work with animals who stop eating early in the experiment.'

The suggestion is that young people who eat very little, but who do consume snacks, soft drinks and confectionery as a large part of their diet, are liable to develop a pathological lack of appetite as the body struggles to avoid vitamin B deficiency states. This applies mainly to young women. Young men rarely eat very little and tend to drink alcoholic drinks, such as beer, that supply as well as leach nutrients. Here, then, is a biochemical account of anorexia which suggests that sometimes anorexia nervosa is accurately labelled the 'slimmer's disease'. The body seeks to avoid illness not by consuming too much energy but by rejecting the toxic food altogether. Lonsdale and Shamberger conclude that the consumption of large quantities of soft drinks is a danger to health not yet identified in the USA and other Western countries, and that eating and drinking a lot of junk food can cause intensely disturbing changes in personality and behaviour which parents, teachers and doctors at the moment label as 'the personality of the growing child or adolescent'.

Apart from old people living alone, students and young office workers are most in danger from deficiency states. Growing boys and girls need significantly more energy from food than adults, both to fuel their bodies' growth and for exercise, games and sport. Adolescents who are not especially active none the less need about 300 more calories of energy from food than they will five years later. A growing mid-teenage boy who plays a lot of football, say, or other sports will be in energy balance at a level of perhaps 4000 calories a day. A girl of the same age who dances at discos three nights a week will require maybe 3000 calories a day.

Many teenagers who consume a lot of junk food are in danger of deficiency states. But usually they are comparatively healthy; they eat nutritious food as well, and do not have enough money, and maybe not the inclination, to smoke or drink a lot, or consume a great deal of junk food. And there is the pressure of the law and parents' disapproval.

## Malaise of young people

At the age of seventeen or eighteen, all this is liable to change—dramatically. When the body stops growing, and if, when they become a student or start work, young people stop taking exercise, they will require perhaps 1000 calories a day less from food. And most of the energy they do need is for the body's basic functions. The only way to be sure of staying healthy when changing, sometimes literally from one month to the next, from a growing active person to an adult sedentary person, is to eat nothing but nutritious food.

And, typically, this is exactly what students and young office workers do not do. No longer obliged to play games, often living away from home for the first time, with parental influence replaced (certainly in the case of students) by often rather ramshackle ways of life, in a milieu where far more drinking and smoking goes on, and with little money, young adults turn to the food that is cheapest and most available.

Students, especially, resist eating institutional food, but rarely have adequate cooking facilities of their own. So there is a sharp rise in the consumption of very energy-heavy foods with high sugar and fat content: chocolate, biscuits, crisps, peanuts with salt, fried food including chips, soft drinks and colas, takeaways, and beer.

A sedentary person cannot burn off the empty energy in these foods, as an active person can. Sedentary adults, accustomed to eating refined sugar, are liable to suffer from being badly nourished, and if they then diet will be in a state of acute malnutrition. But the student or young office worker, whose body is unaccustomed to low energy intakes, and who often eats two or even three times the average amount of junk food, is liable to be in an even worse state. And if such young people then go on a diet, they will be in danger of acute illness, which may take a mental or physical form.

My son Ben, who is just finishing at university, makes a habit of cooking fresh food and even of clearing up after himself. He is regarded with a mixture of awe, puzzlement and derision by the other students and is known by them as 'mother'. I asked him to list the malaises and ailments of his fellow students. These included what is often known as the students' syndrome: depression, confusion, torpor, inability to concentrate, sleeplessness, mood swings, aches and pains, colds, discomfort in the gut, pre-menstrual tension, pallor, sweatiness, and an overriding sense that nothing matters. Sophisticates call all this 'existential angst'. Usually it is not caused by failed love affairs, bad marks or the bomb, but by junk food and refined sugar in particular.

And—the other side of the coin—by lack of fresh food. Take another vitamin, A (carotene). It is found in green and yellow fruit and vegetables, and in liver. It concentrates in the eyes (which is why lack of it causes blindness in extreme situations) and also in the bloodstream and liver. It is attacked by chemical fertilisers present in foods and by air pollution. Symptoms of vitamin A deficiency include bad skin, sensitive eyes, loss of sense of smell, and inability of the nasal membranes to deal with foreign bodies and germs, leading to hay fever and colds.

When I was at university I did not suffer from malaise and ailments. I ate enough nutritive food on top of sugar-heavy foods and gained 2 stone 7 pounds in three years. I stayed healthy by getting fat. Young women at college or in their first jobs often go the other way, staying thin while eating more sugar and so becoming ill for lack of nourishment. Ben has taken another route: he has gained in health at university by eating well and becoming very active physically.

Mothers concerned for the well-being of their children leaving home would do well to ensure that their sons as well as their daughters know what is good food and how to cook good food. Well-nourished students are far less likely to get depressed.

The most popular food sold in Great Britain is saturated with sugar. Market research shows that four of twenty top-selling lines in 1981 were 'all chocolate confectionery', 'chocolate biscuits', 'chocolate filled blocks', and 'sweet biscuits'. Also in the same list were 'potato crisps', 'snack products' (some of which are loaded with fat, some with sugar), 'drinks, carbonated, still, cola'; 'drinks, squashes, cordials' and 'drinks, fruit'.

The energy content of 100 grams of potato is about 80 calories; of an apple, about 40 calories. Many of the most popular foods, however, are heavy with energy—not only fats and flour but also chocolate and sweet biscuits, crisps and sweets. All these are more than five times as dense in energy than potatoes, more than ten times as dense than apples. Cornflakes almost reach this level; other popular cereals, such as Sugar Puffs, which contain 56.5 per cent sugar, have a far denser energy content. Flavoured and fruit yogurts, which have something of a 'health' image, have a sugar content of 17.9 per cent—rather more than digestive biscuits.

It sounds sensational to say that many people in the West are likely to be suffering from minor versions of deficiency diseases, especially when the names of some of the better-known diseases are mentioned—beri-beri, pellagra, scurvy. But most sedentary people in the West are badly nourished; and to say that someone is badly nourished and that they are mal-nourished is to say the same thing. Deficiency diseases are illnesses brought on by malnutrition; and, like obesity and like baldness, deficiency diseases have early, mild stages. These conditions often take the form of malaise and depression of many types.

A rule of thumb for anyone who wants to eat healthy food is: if it's advertised, be careful; if it's canned or packaged, read the label; and if it's got refined sugar in it, don't eat it.

## Refined sugar: the root of much evil

The two vital cores of our bodies and of our health are the alimentary tract, from the mouth and throat to the stomach and through the gut; and the cardiovascular system, of the heart, lungs and blood vessels. One is the means to process food, and the other the means to process oxygen—our two fuels.

In the Third World very many people still suffer and die from the infectious diseases that have largely been conquered in the West by improved sanitation and antibiotics. We in the West suffer and die mostly from the so-called 'degenerative' diseases, principally of the alimentary tract and the cardiovascular system. Some of these diseases—constipation, piles, varicose veins, obstructions and irritations of the gut, hernias, ulcers, gallstones, and diabetes, for example—are inconvenient and can be crippling, but are not usually in themselves fatal. Others—heart disease and cancers—are often deadly. Heart disease is now the biggest killer in Great Britain, the USA and other Western countries.

These diseases are rare, sometimes to the point of being practically unknown, in Third World countries not yet touched by Western influences. They are now known as 'Western diseases' or the 'diseases of civilisation' because they spread wherever Western influence spreads. When Africans come into the towns from the countryside, when Japanese move to Hawaii, when people from the Yemen move to Israel, when Eskimos give up their traditional way of life, when native Americans on reservations accept white life styles, when people in faraway places have an international airport built in the vicinity, then they always begin to suffer and die from the same diseases as Westerners.

Until recently these diseases were generally known as degenerative diseases, because it was believed that they were a consequence of ageing, and that people in the Third World were free of them simply because life outside the Western world was short. A similar argument has sometimes been mounted to explain why so many people in the West get fat whereas people in the Third World living traditional lives as a rule do not; the argument was that Third World people just didn't live long enough.

It is of course true that, in general, life expectancy in Western countries is higher than in the Third World. But life expectancy at the age of 40 is much the same in many non-Western countries as it is in the West; and all countries and societies contain plenty of people who live the Biblical three score years and ten, and longer still. Moreover, many such people have always eaten well, and have not lived very active lives, typically going out to fish or hunt or work in the fields about as often as pre-machine age people did in Western countries. And the fact is that old people in the Third World, living in the country, do not as a rule suffer or die from the so-called 'degenerative' diseases. What then is the cause of these diseases, the scourge of Western societies?

Many doctors who study the incidence of diseases in different societies and different countries agree that the most important single cause of Western diseases is the food we eat, together with our sedentary lives. One doctor who has proposed a causal connection between Western food and Western diseases is Surgeon-Captain J L Cleave, who travelled the world during his professional life in the Royal Navy, studying disease and nutrition patterns in all types of society and maintaining extensive correspondence with other doctors. He published his book *The Saccharine Disease* in 1974, and its impact is still shaking the medical establishment in Britain and the West. Cleave's findings and his thesis have already been hailed as the most important advance in the field of health in this century, together with the discovery of antibiotics.

Cleave's life's work has been to show that the rise in the consumption of processed foods, and the rise in suffering and death from diseases of the alimentary tract and cardiovascular system, which always occur together in Western and Western-influenced countries, are linked. His own name for many of 'the diseases of civilisation' is 'the saccharine disease' because he and now other doctors believe that these diseases are manifestations of one single 'master' disease caused by eating processed foods, and refined sugar in particular.

The causal connection between processed food and Western diseases has been obscured, states Cleave, because of a failure to distinguish between 'the consumption of un-natural, refined carbohydrates, like sugar and white flour, and that of natural, unrefined carbohydrates, like raw and dried fruit and wholemeal flour'.

## Sugar and the gut

Many Western ailments and diseases are of the alimentary tract. It is well known that constipation is caused by a lack of bulk, otherwise known as 'roughage' or fibre, in the food. Eating bran as a supplement to food relieves the condition, which is caused by high-density sugar and other refined carbohydrates. These slow the passage of food through the gut and create hard, compacted stools.

Three other ailments are accelerated by the constant straining itself caused by constipation: hiatus hernia, varicose veins, and piles. All three are uncommon in rural communities in the Third World, where eating large quantities of unrefined carbohydrates containing fibre allows food to pass much more rapidly through the alimentary tract, creating large soft stools.

Cleave proposes that the constant irritation, friction and pressure caused throughout the gut by the difficult passage of the bullet-like material formed from refined sugar and other processed carbohydrate is a prime cause of more serious conditions, such as appendicitis and diverticulosis (a kind of rupture of the colon, very common among middle-aged people in the West). There is also powerful evidence that cancers of the large bowel and colon are caused by the stagnant stool of Western people, containing toxins that cannot be neutralised by the bacteria in the gut. Cleave says:

> The frequency of cancer increases steadily in each successive part of the colon, cancer of the rectum being one of the commonest in the body. It is significant that the irritant effect of any toxins on the intestinal wall must increase steadily in each of these successive parts, both on account of the actual greater production of toxins, and also on account of the progressive slowing that normally occurs in the colonic contents as they pass onwards.

In the nineteenth century it became understood that the irritants in soot caused skin cancer in chimney sweeps. In the last 30 years, it has become accepted that the irritants in cigarette smoke cause cancers of the mouth, tongue, throat, bronchial passages and lungs of smokers, as well as conditions such as bronchitis not in themselves normally deadly. The proposal that refined sugar is a cause of cancer has a similar basis: that the hard and toxic stools formed from food heavy in refined sugar and other processed foods is a constant irritant to the gut, day after day, year after year.

Refined sugar is now universally recognised as the prime cause of tooth decay. The Royal College of Physicians is inclined to accept that refined sugar and other processed foods—'fibre-depleted carbohydrates' as they term them—are also a cause of gallstones. The general conclusion of the Royal College, in their 1980 report on dietary fibre, was a message to food producers, manufacturers and the government to encourage people to 'eat foods which are closer to the natural grain, vegetable or fruit than the highly processed and refined products which now form a large part of our diet'.

Refined sugar has a direct effect on the alimentary tract. Its effect on the cardiovascular system is less direct; and in any case heart disease has several main causes. The silting up of the blood vessels that eventually leads to a heart attack is accelerated by inactivity, by obesity and by diabetic states. Danger signs are high blood pressure; blood high in the dangerous types of fat known as 'low density lipoprotein'; low glucose tolerance; and blood heavy in uric acid or in hormones such as insulin.

## Sugar and heart disease

It is generally accepted nowadays that some of these conditions can be caused by eating a lot of animal fat (also known as 'saturated fat'). Like refined sugar, animal fat is eaten more in the West than in the Third World. It is true that coronary heart disease is uncommon among some peoples who eat a lot of animal meat, such as Eskimos and the Masai. This may be because eventually, after many hundreds of years, the body can adjust to a high level of meat-eating. It is certainly the case that meat eaten from animals that live free is far less fatty than the meat we now eat, from animals that are penned up and cannot be active. It may very well be that the meat we eat in the West is bad for us and causes the build-up of the dangerous low density lipoprotein in the blood simply because it is so fatty. And since fat is very dense in energy, the meat we eat can also contribute to obesity.

But without knowledge of human biochemistry people are liable to believe that eating fat is a bad idea because, well, fat is fat. And as soon as it became common knowledge that heart disease is caused by the build-up of certain types of fat in the blood, dietary fat (meaning, edible fat) became the popular villain. But from the biochemical point of view, any food that causes the danger signs listed above is liable to be a cause of heart disease.

Heart disease is degenerative not in the sense that it is bound to accompany old age but because it takes decades to develop. Cleave made a painstaking study of the rise of heart disease in the

West and showed that, in country after country, this rise was preceded by an acceleration in refined sugar consumption. In Great Britain for example, the great rise in refined sugar consumption almost to today's levels occurred at the end of the nineteenth century, and the great rise in heart disease started to occur 20 years later. Doctors who study the incidence of disease are known as epidemiologists. In the case of refined sugar they have proposed what is known as the 'Rule of 70 and 20', which means that the diseases caused by eating processed foods start to occur in epidemic proportions after the population has been eating at least 70 pounds of refined sugar a year for at least 20 years. Throughout the world this rule holds good.

The clinical work required to back this epidemiological work is now under way. Professor John Yudkin made an early clinical study in the 1960s. He fed high levels of refined sugar to human volunteers and found that 'dietary sucrose can be shown in experiment to produce several of the disturbances that are seen in coronary thrombosis.'

Yudkin is a well-known campaigner against refined sugar, and the sugar manufacturers and their consultants have criticised his results for being inconclusive. What Yudkin found, though, was that after his volunteers had eaten a great deal of refined sugar—far more than they would normally eat—many danger signs started to show themselves: high levels of fat in the blood; low glucose tolerance; and blood heavy in uric acid and in hormones such as insulin, signs of liability to diabetes as well as to heart disease. Yudkin's experiment could not be conclusive; conclusive experiments are normally made on animals and continue until the animal dies, and Yudkin was interested to see what would happen to people after a few weeks of high refined sugar intake. His experiment was a warning.

It is not yet proved that refined sugar is a direct, major cause of heart disease, but the evidence is mounting. Some foods which may well be bad for us are also nutritious, eaten in sensible quantities. But refined sugar has no nourishment in it, and it is absolutely certain that nobody will come to any harm by cutting out eating refined sugar totally. Those of us concerned with our good health may not want to wait until the case against refined sugar is finally proved.

Food manufacturers will be as reluctant to accept the dangers of refined sugar as cigarette manufacturers still are to accept that smoking is deadly. Indeed, the problem with sugar is a bigger one; refined sugar is mixed into every kind of food. And it has only recently been understood that muddling sugar with starch under the general heading of 'carbohydrate' (the reason being that both sugar and starch supply energy to the body) has been a calamity.

The other big confusion about sugar has been the understandable supposition that if natural sugar (in fruit and some vegetables) is good for us, as it surely must be, having been eaten for all of human history, then refined sugar, being chemically a concentrated form of natural sugar, must be good for us too.

The body needs sugar for all its functions. Body sugar is made from carbohydrates, and starchy foods such as cereals, bread, pasta and certain vegetables are as good a source of sugar for the body as are sweet foods. A proper level of blood sugar is essential for physical and mental well-being, and a sandwich or plate of spaghetti a day does indeed help you work, rest and play.

So do the fruits and vegetables containing natural sugar. 'Sugar in Food', the table accompanying this chapter on pages 108–11, lists foods high in natural sugar, which are nutritious. They contain many vitamins and minerals and also the fibre the body needs, as well as energy for the body from sugar.

Refined sugar poisons the body, not because it is sugar, but because it is refined. Other refined foods such as white flour and white rice are also drained of nourishment and cause illness if eaten to the exclusion of nourishing food. Thus a sedentary person who, as well as eating sugar, also eats refined flour in cakes and biscuits makes bad worse. But white flour has some nourishment in it, although far less than wholemeal flour.

One question underlies all other questions about refined sugar. It is simply this. Why, if it is true that sugar is a poison, do we eat it?

Professor Yudkin's answer, that sugar is 'highly palatable', obviously has some truth in it. But why should the body accept the amount of sugar we eat, given that refined sugar has such disastrous effects on our health and well-being? The explanation that sugar is 'highly palatable' seems thin. Another answer, suggested by political radicals such as Hannah Wright of the *New Statesman*, that sugar is cheap, does not rot (being dead), is easily transported, heavily advertised and very profitable obviously has truth in it. In 1979 British press and television advertising for refined sugar and sugar-heavy products totalled £60 million, and advertising works. But this explanation is rather thin, too; a product must be attractive in the first place, before advertising will work. Refined sugar has a magnetism unique among all substances we eat and drink. What is it in refined sugar that overwhelms the body's defences?

The answer lies in the nature of the disease which, after tooth decay, is most unequivocally caused by refined sugar: adult onset diabetes.

### Diabetes

Thomas Willis, the seventeenth-century doctor who first identified diabetes after noting the sweet-smelling urine of his rich patients, wrote in 1685, 'I do much disapprove things preserved or very much seasoned with sugar. I judge the invention of it and its immoderate use to have very much contributed to the vast increase of scurvy in this last age.' Willis did not insist on the causal connection between refined sugar and diabetes with too much vigour. He was court physician to King Charles II, who was enjoying the revenue from the slave trade and from refined sugar. It would not have been tactful for Willis to press his point.

The link between eating great quantities of refined sugar and diabetes is epidemiologically very strong. Summarising various population studies, the Royal College of Physicians wrote in 1980:

A high prevalence of diabetes seems to be characteristic of recently urbanised populations. Examples are Indians and Zulus in South Africa, Yemeni Jews in Israel, American Indians throughout the United States, Maoris in New Zealand, and Polynesians in the Central Pacific island of Nauru. The dietary change which has most often been blamed has been the adoption of refined sugar.

The exploitation of phosphates to be found on Nauru has brought the islanders the highest per capita income in the world. In October 1982 a visiting *Observer* journalist reported that diabetes is epidemic on Nauru. A European nurse reckoned it was about 90 per cent. Dr Thoma, head of medical services, said

We have the second highest rate of diabetes in the world, after the Pima Indians of Phoenix, Arizona. The disease can be prevented and controlled by diet. People here eat too much, and the food is all canned and refined.

Dr Frederick Banting isolated insulin in the 1920s. He regarded it as a palliative, not a cure, for diabetes. He had little doubt about the cause of diabetes in adults. His own observations told Banting that natural sugar is a food but refined sugar is a poison. In 1924 he visited Panama and spoke to a doctor examining men applying for work on the Panama Canal, who had found evidence of diabetes in the urine of two men only—neither of whom proved to be diabetic. Banting commented:

This is the more remarkable because a large percentage of the labourers were natives of Dominica, where a main article of diet was sugar-cane. From the time the children are weaned until they die they eat the sugar-cane. There are also wealthy Spaniards who live in Panama who eat large quantities of refined cane sugar. Indeed much of their food is cooked in syrup. The incidence of diabetes amongst this class is surprisingly high.

Foods containing sugar in its natural state—bananas, apples, grapes and other fruits, sweet potato, onions, carrots and other vegetables and the cane and beet from which refined sugar is made—are nutritious and good for us. The cause of diabetes is not sugar, but sugar in an intensely concentrated form. (It follows that diabetes could develop from eating massive amounts of honey, which in a sense is sugar refined by bees, or dried fruits such as dates, raisins, sultanas and currants. But the body is satisfied by small amounts of these foods, which are dangerous only if eaten by a diabetic.)

The biochemistry of diabetes is easily explained. Sugar is crucial to all the body's functions, and hunger is triggered when the level of sugar in the blood goes below a certain point. Eating any form of carbohydrate raises blood-sugar levels. Carbohydrate eaten in the form of cereals, pasta or bread raises the blood-sugar level, but slowly; as do the sugars in fruit and vegetables, which, bound up with the body of the food when eaten, seep into the bloodstream. The sense of satiety derived from eating such foods is reliable, providing the flour in pastas and bread is wholewheat.

But because of its concentration refined sugar shoots into the bloodstream and is liable to raise it too high. The immediate effect of this sugar rush is very pleasant and is used to good effect in advertisements of products saturated with refined sugar, in which people look happy. But after a certain point, eating refined sugar becomes nauseating: this is especially noticeable if the initial blood-sugar level is very low, as it is in a runner after a long-distance race or a dieter, both of whom feel the need for sugar but can suffer if they eat a candy bar rather than fruit or a sandwich.

For well-being, the level of blood sugar in the body must be neither too low nor too high. When it becomes too high, the body lowers it by releasing insulin from the pancreas into the bloodstream. The faster the blood-sugar level rises, and the higher it goes, the more intense and sudden the reaction of the pancreas. This 'panic' reaction results in too much insulin being poured into the bloodstream, so that, paradoxically, the result of eating or drinking food rich in refined sugar is to change the blood-sugar level from too high to too low. Medically this phenomenon is known as 'rebound hypoglycaemia'. ('Hypo' means low, as 'hyper' means high, and 'glycaemia' refers to the glucose that sugar is turned into in the blood.)

## Low blood sugar

In due course this over-sensitisation of the pancreas leads to a condition which can be termed 'hyperinsulinism' or 'hypoglycaemia', a doctors' term for the whiplash effect of eating and drinking refined sugar or alcoholic drinks, which have the same result. Hypoglycaemia has been much heard about recently, partly because Richard Harris and Julie Andrews have both revealed that they are sufferers, because of alcohol and sweets respectively. As Julie Andrews confessed to *Woman* magazine: 'If I made the foolish mistake of having a brownie when I thought I was going to have an easy day and could indulge myself, I had the most awful fatigue and dizziness. You wouldn't believe it.'

This fatigue and dizziness, together with confusion and depression, can in certain circumstances be very dangerous. The one time I have ever fallen asleep at the wheel was after running a half-marathon after which I ate two chocolate bars for quick energy (this was before I had done the research for this book!). Driving fast down a motorway without any warning I momentarily became unconscious.

Sugar makes you hungry, because sugar in its refined form has the paradoxical effect of lowering blood sugar and setting up a need for the very food that converts quickly into blood sugar—that is, refined sugar. The dependency set up drives out the desire for foods which supply sugar to the body at a natural rate, because that rate comes to feel too slow. Biochemically, the body of someone who eats an average amount of refined sugar alternates from being too high to being too low in blood sugar, and balance is destroyed.

Sugar is with us all the time. It is a term of endearment. It is a comfort. 'The habit of eating for pleasure or comfort such high-energy foods as sweets, chocolates, cakes, biscuits and desserts is initiated in childhood. These items may be given for good behaviour, and withheld as punishment,' points out the Royal College's report on obesity. It goes on to suggest, reasonably enough, that, so trained, adults will turn to such foods when anxious or depressed.

Sugar is one of the things 'little girls are made of'. Babies are kept quiet by sweet water rubbed on their dummies. The new-born infant prefers sugar solution to water. An American study found that:

> Compared with infants not fed sweetened water, the infants fed sweetened water ingested more sucrose solution but not more water at six months of age. Those infants not fed sweetened water exhibited a diminished intake of sucrose solution relative to water at six months of age.

That is to say, give sugar to a tiny baby, and it will learn to want more of it. Children so small that they cannot see over the counter beg the assistant for sweets; and chocolates are a conventional gift for a loved one. In service stations, newspaper shops, supermarket check-outs, sweets are the impulse buy. In Britain the last course at table or in a restaurant, the naughty temptation, is called 'the sweet'. On average, everyone in Britain eats a ton of refined sugar every 20 years. How can it be that refined sugar is so common, so attractive, and yet so bad for us?

### Sweet temptation

Together with alcohol, refined sugar has a special quality that causes the sugar eater to gain fat. Discussions of energy balance tend to treat it like a bank balance: put too much energy in and you get fat, put less energy in and you get thin. People who defend sugar always make a lot of this idea, pointing out that carbohydrates, including sugar, have an energy value of 3.75 calories per gram, compared with 4.1 calories per gram for protein and the much higher figure of 9.3 calories per gram for fat. (The figures are often quoted as 4:4:9, but these are more precise.) The boldest defenders of sugar, such as the British Sugar Bureau, the British publicity organisation for Tate and Lyle and British Sugar, which runs an operation headed by a Member of Parliament from London's Park Lane, go so far as to suggest that sugar is therefore a low-energy food!

Even allowing the accuracy of the bank balance analogy, this argument is specious. People do not eat bars of fat, but they do eat bars of candy; and much of the food we eat that is heavy in fat is made palatable only by the addition of sugar—chocolate bars, ice-cream, cakes and biscuits for example. Most people eat a great deal more sugar than fat, unpalatable by itself.

But the human body is not just a piggy bank for energy from food. The body reacts to different qualities of food in different ways. In the case of refined sugar, a rush of the hormone insulin is provoked, to get rid of the excessively high level of sugar in the blood. The insulin does not 'dissolve' the sugar, as some books suggest. It dumps the blood sugar as fast as possible, by a process that, first, converts the sugar to low-density lipoprotein, the type of fat that is implicated in heart disease, and then, second, converts this fat running free in the blood to fatty tissue.

It follows from this that anyone who is hypoglycaemic because they have consumed refined sugar is in a pre-diabetic state and is liable to gain fat. Refined sugar induces a hormonal reaction from insulin which results in the accumulation of body fat, simply because there is nowhere else in the body the excess blood sugar can go.

It is an error to suppose that diabetes is caused by obesity. An obese person is certainly liable to become diabetic. But in itself obesity is a condition, not a disease, and accompanies the onset of diabetes rather than causing it. Diabetes is triggered when the pancreas is no longer able to release insulin; and the prime cause for this is the continual consumption of refined sugar.

When the pancreas packs up, the process whereby insulin converts sugar in the bloodstream to fat in the blood and then in the body ceases. Instead the sugar is dumped in the kidneys and pours into the urine. It follows, therefore, that weight loss, or failure to continue to gain weight, is a sign that a pre-diabetic condition has become diabetes. And this is indeed what happens. Dr James Anderson, Professor of Medicine at the University of Kentucky, states: 'Although adult-type diabetics are usually overweight they sometimes seem to lose a little weight before they are first treated by a doctor.'

Anyone who consumes more energy than their body needs will gain fat. But refined sugar makes you fat not only because, being concentrated, it is dense in energy, but also, and most important, because it disturbs the hormone insulin. Sedentary or even moderately active people who eat an average amount of refined sugar, or who drink a lot of alcohol, face one of two dismal futures. Either they will eat enough nutritious food, and sugar as well, in which case they will end up overweight or obese, and quite likely suffer from diabetes, heart and other diseases in middle age. Or they will avoid gaining weight by eating maybe only half the nutritious food their body needs, in which case the result will be malaise, debilitation and, eventually, chronic deficiency states—the junk food syndrome.

### Sugar addiction

But if sugar is deadly, why do our bodies accept it? What is the overwhelming attraction of sugar? The answer is in front of our eyes every day, in service stations, newspaper shops, supermarkets and restaurants. Imagine the reaction of a child refused sweets, or of adults told there is no sugar for their tea or coffee. The child will make a fuss; may even filch money to buy sweets, or steal the sweets from the shop. The adults will fidget; may refuse the drink, and be pleased if you borrow a cup of sugar from a neighbour. Such behaviour is so usual and expected that we do not realise how striking and strange it is. The mother distrusts her child, and why? Because the child has stolen pennies from her purse. And what for? To buy sweets.

The Department of Health and Social Security, in an official document published in 1975, had this to say:

Better dental health could be assured if only parents discouraged children from eating sweets, lollipops, drinks containing sugar and so on . . . but a childhood without sweets may well be regarded by many as a fate worse than an adulthood without teeth.

If refined sugar were unknown and were now introduced, and its effects observed, it would be made illegal. We shy away from the word 'addictive', tending to use it only of substances which, as well as being poisonous, are illegal. But, after all, it was only 200 years ago that mothers quietened their babies by means of opium smeared on a little finger. Later, opium became illegal.

We crave sugar. That should be clue enough. We speak jokingly of being 'sugar junkies' and wanting a 'sugar hit', and jokes are always clues. A substance is addictive when it drives out a natural body function, replacing it with an artificial function on which the body then comes to depend. Smoking, for example, is addictive for two separate reasons. The carbon monoxide in tobacco smoke inhibits the flow of oxygen to the blood, and the nicotine in tobacco inhibits the flow of hormones known as endorphins, the body's natural pain-killers. The craving for cigarettes after giving up smoking is not 'just in the mind'; the body learns to crave carbon monoxide and nicotine.

Likewise, refined sugar overwhelms the body's natural reaction to the sugar within fruit or the starch in vegetables and cereals. Eating refined sugar causes an artificially high blood-sugar level; then, because of the body's defence system, an artificially low blood-sugar level; and so a craving for sugar. As Mr Mars discovered, eating one Mars Bar creates the habit for another Mars Bar.

## Table 1. Sugar in Food

It is not easy to avoid eating refined sugar. This table is designed to help you. Foods heavy in refined sugar are included in the first list. The top part, of foods containing more than 40 per cent refined sugar, is mostly confectionery; but some sweet breakfast cereals such as Sugar Puffs are not much more than vehicles for refined sugar. The middle part of the list, of foods containing more than 20 per cent refined sugar, includes some items tasting fairly savoury or thought of as 'health' foods, such as sweet pickle, rich tea biscuits and packet muesli. The bottom part of the list is a small selection of foods containing more than 5 per cent refined sugar. Note the fruit salad: fruits canned in syrup are 15 to 25 per cent refined sugar. Almost all breakfast cereals have added refined sugar. Soft drinks such as Coca-Cola are basically water, refined sugar and flavourings. Almost all canned food has added refined sugar: look at the label.

Refined sugar supplies nothing but energy. The second list is of foods high in natural sugar, which also contain many nutrients. While honey and dried fruit are both nutritious, it is better to eat them sparingly and not as a substitute for refined sugar. Fruit juice has more natural sugar than the fruit itself, the fibrous content having been removed; prefer the whole fruit.

The body needs sugar for energy, but you do not have to eat food containing sugar. Starch converts to sugar in the body just as readily as dietary sugar. The third list is designed as a means to wean you off refined sugar; it is a selection of dairy products, fruits and vegetables, cereals and other foods containing little or no sugar.

*Foods High in Refined Sugar*

| | per cent | | per cent |
|---|---|---|---|
| Sugar (white, brown) | 100.0 | Muesli (packaged) | 26.2 |
| Peppermints | 100.0 | Fruit salad (canned)[1] | 25.0 |
| Meringues | 95.6 | Tomato ketchup | 22.9 |
| Boiled sweets | 86.9 | Ice-cream | 22.6 |
| Golden syrup | 79.0 | Rich tea biscuits | 22.3 |
| Drinking chocolate (dry) | 73.8 | Malt loaf | 18.6 |
| Toffees | 70.0 | Fruit yogurt[1] | 17.9 |
| Jam, marmalade | 69.0 | Digestive biscuits | 16.4 |
| Mars Bar | 65.8 | All–Bran | 15.4 |
| Ribena (undiluted) | 60.0 | Doughnuts | 15.0 |
| Chocolate (plain) | 59.5 | Jelly (water) | 14.2 |
| Chocolate (milk) | 56.5 | Currant buns | 14.0 |
| Sugar Puffs | 56.5 | Salad cream | 13.4 |
| Bounty bar | 53.7 | Flavoured yoghurt[1] | 13.0 |
| Bournvita (dry) | 52.0 | Coca-Cola | 10.5 |
| Horlicks (dry) | 49.4 | Lucozade | 9.0 |
| Fruit cake | 46.7 | Rice Krispies | 9.0 |
| Wafers (filled) | 44.7 | Canned sweetcorn[1] | 8.9 |
| Chocolate biscuits | 43.4 | Cornflakes | 7.4 |
| Ginger nuts | 35.8 | Crispbread, Energen | 7.4 |
| Jam, treacle tart | 33.6 | Peanut butter | 6.7 |
| Branston pickle | 32.6 | Weetabix | 6.1 |
| Sponge cake | 30.5 | Tomato soup (condensed; diluted) | 5.6 |
| Rusks (for babies) | 30.0 | Orange, lemonade (diluted) | 5.6 |
| Chocolate digestive biscuits | 28.5 | Baked beans | 5.2 |

[1] including small amount of natural sugar content

*Foods High in Natural Sugar*

| | per cent | | per cent |
|---|---|---|---|
| Honey[1] | 76.0 | Plums, damsons | 9.6 |
| Sultanas, raisins | 64.5 | Figs (fresh) | 9.5 |
| Dates (dried) | 63.9 | Orange juice | 9.5 |
| Currants | 63.1 | Sweet potato (boiled) | 9.1 |
| Figs (dried) | 52.9 | Peaches | 9.1 |
| Milk (skimmed, dried)[2] | 52.8 | Oranges[3] | 8.5 |
| Apricots (dried) | 43.4 | Spring onions | 8.5 |
| Prunes (dried) | 40.3 | Damsons (stewed) | 8.1 |
| Milk (dried)[2] | 39.4 | Tangerines | 8.0 |
| Prunes (stewed) | 20.4 | Horseradish (raw) | 7.3 |
| Bananas | 16.2 | Chestnuts | 7.0 |
| Lychees (raw) | 16.0 | Apricots (raw) | 6.7 |
| Grapes, white[3] | 15.3 | Blackcurrants | 6.6 |
| Mangoes | 15.3 | Coconut (dessicated) | 6.4 |
| Grapes, black[3] | 13.0 | Blackberries | 6.4 |
| Apple juice | 13.0 | Strawberries | 6.2 |
| Nectarines | 12.4 | Passion fruit | 6.2 |
| Cherries | 11.9 | Apricots (stewed) | 5.6 |
| Apples (raw)[3] | 11.8 | Raspberries | 5.6 |
| Greengages | 11.8 | Carrots (raw) | 5.4 |
| Pineapple[3] | 11.6 | Grapefruit[3] | 5.3 |
| Pomegranates (juice) | 11.6 | Melons | 5.3 |
| Pears[3] | 10.6 | Onion (raw) | 5.2 |
| Onions (fried) | 10.1 | Chick peas, dahl | 5.2 |
| Beetroot (cooked) | 9.9 | Plums (stewed) | 5.2 |

[1] honey has nutrients but in a sense is refined (by bees)

[2] lactose

[3] juice from these fruits has 1 to 2 per cent more sugar

*Foods Low in Sugar*

| | per cent | | per cent |
|---|---|---|---|
| Fresh milk[1] | 4.7 | Cucumbers | 1.8 |
| Natural yogurt[1] | 4.6 | Corn on the cob | 1.7 |
| Leeks (boiled) | 4.6 | Brussels sprouts | 1.6 |
| Almonds | 4.3 | Puffed wheat | 1.5 |
| Carrots (boiled) | 4.2 | Butter beans | 1.5 |
| Coconut | 3.7 | Runner beans | 1.3 |
| Peas (canned)[2] | 3.6 | Marrow | 1.3 |
| Loganberries | 3.4 | Lettuce | 1.2 |
| Crispbread, Ryvita[2] | 3.2 | Spinach | 1.2 |
| Tomato juice | 3.2 | Celery | 1.2 |
| Lemons | 3.2 | Pastry | 1.0 |
| Peanuts | 3.1 | Cauliflower | 0.8 |
| Aubergines | 2.9 | Lentils | 0.8 |
| Gooseberries (stewed) | 2.9 | Spaghetti, pastas | 0.8 |
| Tomatoes | 2.8 | Potatoes | 0.6 |
| Parsnips (boiled) | 2.7 | Watercress | 0.6 |
| Tomato soup[2] | 2.6 | Shredded wheat | 0.4 |
| Vegetable soup[2] | 2.5 | Olives | Trace |
| Water biscuits | 2.3 | Rice | Trace |
| Instant potato[2] | 2.2 | Porridge | Trace |
| White cabbage (boiled) | 2.2 | Tea | Trace |
| White bread, rolls[2] | 2.0 | Artichokes | 0 |
| Wholewheat bread[2] | 2.0 | Mushrooms | 0 |
| Peas (fresh) | 1.8 | Meat, fish | 0 |
| Avocado pears | 1.8 | Marmite | 0 |

[1] Lactose. Yogurt also has a little galactose

[2] Refined sugar

Chief source of information: *McCance and Widdowson's The Composition of Foods* edited by A A Paul and D A T Southgate (HMSO 1978).

# CHAPTER FOUR

# Swallow It Whole

The word 'health' in English is based on an Anglo-Saxon word 'hale' meaning 'whole': that is, to be healthy is to be whole. Likewise, the English 'holy' is based on the same root as 'whole'. All of this indicates that man has sensed always that wholeness or integrity is an absolute necessity to make life worth living.
DAVID BOHM
*Wholeness and the Implicate Order*

We always had plenty, our children never cried from hunger, neither were our people in want. The rapids of Rock River furnished us with an abundance of excellent fish, and the land being very fertile never failed to produce good crops of corn, beans, pumpkins, and squashes. If a prophet had come to our village in those days and told us that the things were to take place which have since come to pass, none of our people would have believed him.
BLACK HAWK, CHIEF OF THE SOUK AND FOX
in *Touch the Earth*, by T C McLuhan

### More diet memoirs

In my dieting days, I carried around a leaflet called the 'Unit Eating Guide' whose introduction promised:

An evolutionary approach . . . to the problem of correct eating. No longer will you be able to say you feel hungry. This is because a very wide variety of foods can be freely taken at any time.

Ah! Magic! A diet that didn't involve cutting calories! No wonder I picked it up. The principle of this system was to concentrate the mind of the dieter on the monster carbohydrate: 'Keep your carbohydrate consumption down to a low level by taking little of the carbohydrate foods, but as much as you like of the non-carbohydrate foods.'

It was a handy little guide; it listed foods in three groups. Group A was 'eat as much as you like'. It included:

| | | | |
|---|---|---|---|
| Duck | Cockles | Butter | Cabbage |
| Black pudding | Cod | Cream cheese | Courgettes |
| Faggots | Flathead | Processed cheese | Okra |
| Lard | Jewfish | Cream | Olives |
| Liver paste | Leather jacket | Margarine | Pumpkin |
| Suet | Oysters | Cooking oil | Ginger |
| Tripe | Pollack | Salad oil | Gravy |

Group C was printed on red paper. Looking at the leaflet now, I well recall the feelings I had as I peered down the list of the foods which, I was being led to believe, were making me into Michelin Man. 'Danger! Avoid if possible!' was printed on top of this list, rather like the road signs that warn you of falling rocks. The list of baddies included:

| | | | |
|---|---|---|---|
| Ale | Flour | Macaroni | Sugar |
| All-Bran | Fructose | Oatmeal | Taro |
| Bread (brown) | Gin | Plum pudding | Teff |
| Bread (white) | Grapes | Port | Vermicelli |
| Cereals | Honey | Potato | Yam |
| Bun | Horlicks | Ryvita | Yogurt (flavoured) |
| Chocolate | Ice-cream | Sago | Yorkshire pudding |

There was a time when I knew these lists more or less off by heart. Their alphabeticisation did hold a certain appeal. Meals of toffees, tonic water, treacle and vermicelli were Out. Menus of garfish, groper, gurnet and haddock were In; as were schnapper, seaslugs, shrimps and skate, or mayonnaise, mustard, pepper and pickles. I wondered, eyeing the oysters in the fishmongers, which fish was the leather jacket. I believed that if, in a cafe, I was told, 'Sorry, love, taro and teff are off,' I was missing nothing that would do me any good.

'One thing you will notice from the examples we have given, the foods you can eat are quite straight-forward ordinary foods, and you can eat them whenever you like,' said the guide. The main warning in the introduction was against the red foods in group C. These were, it said, 'foods that are rich in carbohydrate, and don't contain much in the way of nutrients'. The guide was put out in 1972.

### The confusion of starch with sugar

Dr Irwin Stillman's *Doctor's Quick Weight Loss Diet* was popular at about the same time. One of the diets he recommends is the 'HF-HP' diet. 'The usual basic restriction at its strongest may be summed up in one sentence: don't touch carbohydrates, sugar, salt, fruits, cereals, bread, rice, potatoes, alcohol.'

Not only don't eat or drink—don't touch. The inference was not only that carbohydrates made you fat but that they could give you typhoid. Richard Mackarness, a psychiatrist, wrote *Eat Fat and Grow Slim* which, its publishers claim, has sold over a million copies. While warning against sugar and refined foods, Mackarness says:

> Try to develop a carbohydrate alarm system, so that whenever you are confronted with a food which does or even *might* contain carbohydrate, a little bell goes off in your head and you avoid the temptation to eat it.

Unclean! Unclean! 'The first thing to realise', writes Dr Mackarness 'is that it is carbohydrate (starch and sugar) and carbohydrate only, which fattens fat people.'

The Consumers' Association is also enthusiastic about low-carbohydrate diets, as an alternative to diets that cut calories. In *Which? Way to Slim*, published in 1978, the authors say:

The foods which are richest in carbohydrate are, on the whole, the ones which are poorest in proteins, vitamins and minerals . . . . The low carbohydrate diet is therefore particularly suitable for growing children.

Much like my 'Unit Eating Guide' and Dr Mackarness, *Which?* says of carbohydrate-rich food: 'Think of it as a traffic light. The red light means STOP for the things to avoid . . . .' And the list includes bread, breakfast cereals, biscuits, flour, honey, nuts, potatoes, spaghetti, sugar and sweets. In the section on staying slim after following the low-carbohydrate method, *Which?* lets the slimmer-pilgrim know that she is on a long, stony road. A cartoon shows a housewife polishing a sideboard, eyeing a plate of biscuits with a red 'X' through them. The text says:

By following the low-carbohydrate method, you had to cut right down on sweet and starchy foods. If you have managed to do this successfully while you were losing weight, you may well be happy never to see a chocolate or potato again. Your only danger then would be eating too much protein and fat which would supply too many calories.

The basic message, though, is that the baddies are sugar and starch, bracketed together as carbohydrates.

*Vogue* magazine has followed the same line for many years. In the 1960s it said: 'The simplest do-it-yourself answer is—we're sorry to say—some kind of crash diet. It's human nature to want quick results so, for quick returns, cut out starch and sugar.'

In 1966 *Vogue* produced a Peanut Diet, 'devised by one of Britain's leading nutrition consultants'. 'Forbidden foods include everything made with flour or cornflour, root vegetables, peas, beans, cereals, pastas, all sugar, sweets, sweetened drinks.' The dieter is told to replace one of the main meals of the day with 2 oz of peanuts (with salt) and also an orange.

The *Vogue Book of Diets and Exercise*, published in 1980, lists various low-carbohydrate diets, including one recommended by Edgar S Gordon, Professor of Medicine at the University of

Wisconsin, one created for the late Aga Khan (a man not noted for a slim figure) and one by Robert Atkins, of *Dr Atkins' Diet Revolution* and *Dr Atkins' Nutrition Breakthrough*. No peanuts, says Dr Atkins. And, in the Jove-like style he shares with Dr Stillman, Dr Tarnower and all the most effective salesmen, prophetic, fatherly, threatening, he says:

> Super Don'ts. Put these out of your life (and your recipes). Bread, cereal, corn, ice-cream, ketchup, macaroni, milk, potatoes, pulse vegetables, rice, spaghetti, sugar, sweets/chewing gum, water biscuits. Note: one piece of chewing gum can spoil the whole chemical balance.

Until Audrey Eyton's *F-Plan Diet*, the best-selling diet book in Great Britain was Professor John Yudkin's *This Slimming Business*, first published in 1958. Yudkin is best known professionally for his hostility to refined sugar. But in his writings for the general public, dieters in particular, this hostility is extended to all carbohydrates. He is an author and writer of numerous articles (sometimes under a *nom de plume*) for periodicals, and a nutrition consultant; and he has probably done more than any other nutritionist to have us believe that carbohydrates are, for the slimmer, the villain.

Yudkin's theory of nutrition is that the food eaten by our hunter-gatherer ancestors was meat, fish, roots, berries, fruit, leaves, rich in protein and also fat, but including little carbohydrate. On this theory, he gives us a model to follow, a 'Stone Age Diet': 'The nearer we get to man's hunting and food gathering diet, the more likely we are to be well-nourished, and the more we can depend on our instinctive choice.' Yudkin sees agriculture as a snare. The discovery of cereals encouraged settlement and the beginning of civilisation. The agriculturist's food is chiefly composed of carbohydrate and contains less protein and fat than that of the hunter-gatherer. And, Yudkin concludes, in a passage which in effect provides the intellectual underpinning for all low-carbohydrate diets: 'My theory is that this is the fundamental fault with the diets of civilisation.' He then goes on to set out his system of 'carbohydrate units', explaining that all the dieter need do is memorise a long list of carbohydrate-rich foods.

My 'Unit Eating Guide' also used the carbohydrate unit system. I got it from a doctor who prescribed the slimming drug 'Ponderax'. The Guide is given free to doctors, worldwide, by Servier Laboratories, manufacturers of Ponderax, which is promoted as the one slimming drug that is not addictive. Servier estimate that they have produced 250,000 copies of the Guide, which is now in wall-chart form. Servier's nutritional consultant is Professor John Yudkin.

Not so much is heard nowadays of low-carbohydrate diets, but carbohydrate remains accused of being the guilty food. In his report *Sweet Nothings*, Aubrey Sheiham points out the systematic confusion between starch and sugar which publications issued to the British public still perpetrate. The British Medical Association's *You and Your Baby*, produced for mothers in 1977, says: 'Do eat sensibly. It means eating little carbohydrate.' Boots produced a leaflet for expectant mothers in 1975. It says: 'Potatoes, bread, sugar, cakes and biscuits are carbohydrates. They provide energy and warmth, but should only be taken sparingly.'

Professor Yudkin is also consultant to the National Dairy Council, whose *Keeping Fit in Retirement* says: 'If you want to lose some weight, cut out or reduce some of the "starchy" foods you eat. These are bread, cakes, pastry, sugar, jam, rice, biscuits, cereals and potatoes.'

Ironically, given Yudkin's hostility to refined sugar, his own argument that starch and sugar are equally objectionable is turned on its head by the sugar manufacturers, who argue that sugar and starch are equally desirable. The British Sugar Bureau, the publicity organisation for Tate and Lyle and British Sugar, published *Questions and Answers on Sugar* in 1977, circulating it free to NHS and private doctors, to doctors and surgeons in hospitals, to health education officers, 1224 registered dieticians and 600 medical correspondents of the national press and women's magazines. I first came across it on the shelves of the

Health Education Council's library. *Questions and Answers* says that refined sugar is a

> carbohydrate which is easily absorbed and enables the body to replace lost energy quickly. This property is appreciated by athletes, sportsmen, busy mothers and active growing children . . . . Our calorie needs are provided by balanced meals containing protein, carbohydrates, including starches and sugars, and fats. When weight reduction is indicated most dieticians support an overall reduction in food intake.

Everybody who has been on a low-carbohydrate diet will recognise the language used to make the dieter conform. 'Danger!' 'Try to develop a carbohydrate alarm system.' 'Think of it as a traffic light.' '. . . the whole chemical balance'. 'Should be taken only sparingly.' The metaphors and images buzz around the brain of the bemused dieter, who is invited to think of carbohydrates as an abyss, a sin, oncoming traffic, a toxin, or a medicine. Always, though, the dieter is told to distrust his or her own body; and women are especially susceptible to this message.

British housewives were asked in a survey to name the foods that should be avoided when slimming. Expressed as the percentage of housewives naming each food, the eight foods most often named were:

| | | | |
|---|---|---|---|
| Potatoes | 62% | Starches | 22% |
| Bread | 55% | Sweets | 16% |
| Sugar | 31% | Fat | 10% |
| Cakes | 25% | Carbohydrate | 7% |

Biscuits, pastry, fried food and butter came further down the list. In the minds of slimmers and would-be slimmers sugars and starches are mingled together. For the last 20 years and more, British mothers, children, dieters, pensioners, doctors, dieticians, nutritionists, health educators, nurses, journalists, and readers of newspapers, magazines and books have been taught, systematically, to think of carbohydrates as bad food and to think of sugars and starches, both of which are carbohydrates, as equally bad. In their publicity the sugar manufacturers reinforce this message, proposing that sugars and starches, both being carbohydrates, are equally good.

## The medical revolution for the 1980s

All this is changing now, and the change is so radical that it requires explanation. In 1977 a committee of the United States Senate, under the chairmanship of George McGovern, published a report, *Dietary Goals for The United States*. The report made a sharp distinction between sugar and starch, recommending that consumption of sugar be more than halved and also that consumption of the hitherto despised starch be more than doubled, as follows:

|         | *Total energy intake %* | |
|---------|------|-------------|
|         | 1977 | Recommended |
| Protein | 12   | 12          |
| Fat     | 42   | 30          |
| Starch  | 22   | 48          |
| Sugar   | 24   | 10          |
| Total   | 100  | 100         |

The McGovern committee was concerned with the health of US citizens, and with obesity in particular. The Royal College of Physicians, in their 1983 report on obesity, likewise stated that foods rich in starch are not fattening and are also healthy:

> The public and many in the medical profession have come to consider dietary carbohydrates as being particularly conducive to weight gain and the development of obesity, no distinction being made between sucrose (sugar) and starch as sources of dietary carbohydrate.

In common with the twenty-three young men of Galway, Lord Byron lost weight on a potato diet. The Royal College indicates why: 'These views on the fattening qualities of dietary carbohydrates are mistaken, and it can be argued that low carbohydrate diets are inappropriate on general nutritional grounds.'

The Royal College agree with the McGovern committee that fat intake should fall to 30 per cent of total energy intake and also that intake of refined sugar should be halved. 'The old concept of reducing only total carbohydrates is nutritionally and medically inappropriate, since there is increasing evidence that fibre-rich starchy foods are important components of the diet.'

One by one, countries all over the developed world are now issuing recommendations along these lines. The story behind this radical new view of the relationship between certain types of food and obesity, illness and health is the story of a group of British doctors who are having the same impact on medicine that Darwin had on science and Keynes had on economics.

These doctors have put a time-bomb under the conventional Western medicine of drugs and surgery. They are in course of proving beyond reasonable doubt that many of the most common Western diseases can only be checked by conventional medical treatment, and are caused by what we eat and do not eat. These non-infectious diseases can therefore be prevented. Between now and the end of the century Western medicine is likely to experience the biggest change ever in its history—towards prevention. This movement will be encouraged by citizens who are appalled by the effects of drugs and who, by taking responsibility for themselves, will encourage doctors to practise the medicine of health rather than illness.

### The value of wholefood

In telling the story of this medical revolution, I am in debt to Dr Hugh Trowell, originator of the concept of 'Western diseases', who has shown me the first chapter of his forthcoming book, *Dietary Fibre, Refined Carbohydrate Foods and Disease*, to be published by Academic Press in 1984.

So far the thesis of this book, for people who want to lose fat and for people who want to gain health, amounts to two don'ts. Do not go on a diet, and do not eat processed, 'refined', sugar. The rest of this chapter is concerned with good food—with the unrefined, starchy carbohydrates that have been wrongly blamed as a cause of fatness, wrongly condemned as of little nutritional value, and that are now rightly championed as the staff of life.

Surgeon-Captain J L Cleave, the British doctor who more than any other has exposed the role of refined sugar in Western diseases, is also an advocate of unprocessed carbohydrate. Cleave has pointed out that the danger of carbohydrates does not lie in their energy content, which is low in their natural state as cereal, beans, vegetables and some fruits, but in their refined, concentrated state:

> It is perfectly true that the calories in, for example an apple, are much the same as those in a teaspoonful of sugar, and therefore at first sight the danger in cases of obesity would appear to be the same in each. But there is an enormous difference between the two in one vital respect—the amount a person needs to consume of each before the appetite is appeased. A person may over-consume sugar very easily—but not apples.

For Cleave the difference between eating refined sugar and eating apples (including natural sugar) is the one between craving and satisfaction, between obesity and no obesity.

Since Cleave began his pioneering work, other British doctors have emphasised not only the dangers of refined sugar but also—and to a considerable extent this is the reverse side of the same coin—the benefits of dietary fibre. Fibre is that part of food derived from the cellular walls of plants such as sugar cane. In effect it is the skeleton of the plant. It is of course discarded in the refining process. Humans digest little of it, and until recently therefore nutritionists and doctors assumed that fibre had no value as food.

The identification of the value of dietary fibre has been principally a British achievement, a result, as Dr Hugh Trowell has explained to me, of the British 'having colonies where doctors could study the changing incidence of disease in time and in place and in various groups over a period of several years. History and geography favoured us.'

Sir Robert McCarrison was Director of Research on Nutrition in India, then part of the British Empire, in the 1920s. He was impressed by the superb health and physique of the people of the state of Hunza in northernmost India, 'whose sole food to this day consists of grains, vegetables, and fruits, with a certain amount of milk and butter, and meat only on feast days'. Although they dwelt in primitive and harsh conditions, the Hunza in McCarrison's day were long-lived, and their illnesses were wholly unconnected with food. By contrast, McCarrison deplored the state of health of European people, fed on processed food. 'Green vegetables are scanty, and such as there are, are often cooked to the point of almost complete extraction of their vitamin content and salts. White bread has largely replaced wholemeal bread.' And he noted that a drop in infant and adult mortality accompanied the national canteens established in Belgium during the First World War and the consumption of large quantities of whole cereals and potatoes in Denmark during the same war. Ironically, shortages forced the Danes to eat this healthy food; in peacetime cattle and swine ate the cereals and potatoes.

In his book *Nutrition and Health*, McCarrison also quoted studies by Dr G E Friend, of special interest to me because Friend was the doctor—before my time—at my own school, Christ's Hospital. I well remember, in the 1950s, eating Prewett's wholewheat and 'squashed fly' biscuits (the latter named after the dried fruit they contained), the remnants of the doctor's campaign against refined food. Alas, the boys of my generation tended to flick Mr Prewett's good food at each other, like miniature frisbees. They were effective missiles. We preferred to eat sugary biscuits from our tuck lockers, having no idea of Dr Friend's principles: 'The deficiency of white bread in Vitamin B1 is one of the most serious dietary deficiencies to which our populations are being subjected at the present time.'

## Health in black Africa and during wars

Dr Alec Walker, who left Great Britain for South Africa in 1938, has extended McCarrison's work. Dr Walker has studied the changes in eating habits and disease patterns in black Africans who have moved from rural to urban areas and in Indians moving from rural India to urban South Africa. He has found that the move into urban areas reduced the life expectancy of middle-aged Africans and Indians. In 1974 he reported that the expectation of life of South African blacks aged 50 exceeded that of whites of the same age. In rural India people of 50 usually died of infectious diseases and had a 14.5 per cent chance of reaching the age of 70; in South Africa they usually died of coronary heart disease, strokes, cancer or diabetes and had only a 9 per cent chance of reaching 70. At an older age the differences are even more remarkable: 'allowing for differences in population numbers, there are at least 20 times more Bantu over 100 years old than whites.'

Dr Denis Burkitt, who worked for 30 years as a surgeon in East Africa, also observed that Africans living in rural areas did not get fat:

In the 1920s doctors in East Africa reported that almost every African was slim. Even the soldiers who were liberally fed with traditional African food rarely appeared obese. In contrast urban Africans are commonly obese today and some of the overweight rulers are familiar figures on news media.

Like Dr Burkitt, Dr Walker became convinced that rural Africans and Indians who moved to urban areas began to suffer from obesity, and die from Western diseases, because their eating habits changed. Their traditional food, like the traditional food of virtually everybody in the world before the spread of industrialisation in the West, was mainly composed of whole grain, rich in starch, fibre and other nutrients, lightly processed and lightly—if at all—cooked, together with vegetables and fruit. But in the urban areas they ate sugar and fat instead of starch, and fewer vegetables. The dramatic difference was the virtual elimination of dietary fibre.

Dr Hugh Trowell was the first person to identify 'Western diseases' as such. He worked in the same large teaching hospital in Uganda as Dr Burkitt. His book *Non-infectious Diseases in Africa*, proposed that fibre gives protection against various diseases of the lower gut and bowel, was published in 1960; and sold twenty-seven copies in its first year. Undaunted, Trowell, with Burkitt, later identified seventeen diseases of previously uncertain origin that are common in the West and sent the list to thirty-four doctors working in teaching hospitals all over the world. Their response confirmed that these diseases were rare among hunter-gatherers, uncommon among peasants, but common among people with Western food habits who take little exercise and smoke a lot.

Dr Cleave was independently accumulating his own evidence against refined sugar and in favour of unrefined starch. In the Second World War, enemy attacks on Allied convoys reduced supplies of wheat to Great Britain from the USA. The government therefore stipulated that bread should be made from 86 per cent whole wheat. The 'National Loaf' was the staple food from 1941 to 1954, when restrictions were lifted and the white loaf most people eat today was introduced. Cleave points out that between 1941 and 1954 mortality from diabetes fell by 54 per cent, a finding similar to Sir Robert McCarrison's in the previous war.

The people of Singapore, faced with acute food shortages before the island fell to the Japanese in 1942, were compelled by the British authorities to eat brown rice, simply because the process of refining and polishing rice resulted in 30 out of every 100 tons of unprocessed grain being discarded. After one year of this regime infant mortality fell by half.

Cleave made two more remarkable discoveries in the Second World War. His brother, Surgeon-Captain H L Cleave, was a prisoner of war of the Japanese and the surgeon in charge of British prisoners in Hong Kong and later in Tokyo. British prisoners who worked on the Burma railway were fed whole, brown rice and bran normally fed to swine. They did not suffer from ulcers. In Hong Kong, prisoners were fed processed white rice; ulcers were common. The same prisoners were then transferred to Tokyo and fed brown rice; the ulcers vanished. Ulcers are often blamed on stress. But the ulcer-free prisoners in Tokyo were being held in a city that was largely destroyed by American bombing.

J L Cleave himself corresponded extensively with Germans who served and were made prisoner on the Russian Front. To the astonishment of German doctors in the front line, the closer their soldiers came to the Russians in the Stalingrad campaign, and the more anxiety, cold and fatigue they suffered, the fewer ulcers they had. The reason, Cleave came to realise, was that over-extended supply lines forced the soldiers to forage for food. They ate frozen raw vegetables, turnips in particular, and sour wholemeal bread. One ex-prisoner wrote to Cleave:

> Our bread in the Russian camps did not consist of refined flour, but of unrefined wheat, rye, barley or maize, with frequently up to 20 per cent of peas, beans or soya bean. We were fed the Russian way. Cabbage soup played a dominant part.

While in captivity the Germans ate little animal protein, animal fat or refined sugar. They had no ulcers. After repatriation to Germany, many of those who had ulcers before the Russian campaign suffered relapses.

More recently, in a study of 337 middle-aged men in London, Professor Jeremy Morris of the London School of Hygiene and Tropical Medicine found that men least subject to certain types of heart disease were those who ate most wholewheat bread and breakfast cereal, most vegetable (as opposed to animal) fat, and whose energy intake from food was highest. The men most liable to heart attacks ate the least amount of starchy food.

During the 1970s Dr Trowell, with colleagues, found that fibre-rich food is a protection against dangerous levels of fats in the blood, different forms of heart disease, and diabetes, as well as obesity. Contrary to previous practice, diabetics were—and now are—taken off drugs and put on therapeutic diets of starchy food including fibre, which worked. The culmination of Dr Trowell's research was the publication of the Royal College of Physicians' report *Medical Aspects of Dietary Fibre* in 1980 which, with some qualifications, supported his work. McCarrison and Walker, Cleave, Burkitt, Trowell and others believe that lack of dietary fibre is an important cause of Western diseases of the alimentary tract, and also of the cardiovascular system and vital organs. Their thesis is now becoming established throughout the West. It is a thesis of fundamental importance to modern medicine, because it puts the emphasis on prevention and the responsibility for prevention in the hands of the individual citizen. That is why Dr Trowell and his colleagues are creating a revolution in medicine.

## The value of fibre

The action of dietary fibre is principally not that of a nutrient but that of an essential package for nutrients. Its effect is the opposite of that of foods whose fibre has been 'refined' out of them, and of sugar in particular. The passage of fibrous foods through the upper alimentary tract is relatively slow. And because fibre is indigestible, it surrounds the nutrients with which it is bound, enabling them to be released into the bloodstream in a sustained manner, not in a rush. Starch, the carbohydrate bound with fibre in the form of wholewheat bread, can therefore raise the blood-sugar level at a natural speed, without provoking the insulin response that refined sugar causes. Likewise, the natural sugars, and also the carbohydrates, in fruit are released into the bloodstream slowly. (Fruit juices and even fruit purees, while not provoking an insulin response as violent as that of refined sugar, can nevertheless have this effect; the whole fruit is to be preferred.)

The bulk of fibrous food provides the intestinal muscle with the work it was designed to do, and the passage of fibre-rich food through the lower intestinal tract is comparatively faster. The fibre survives to enter the large bowel and there absorbs acids which without the presence of fibre become toxic, creating irritation and eventually the risk of cancers. If fibre is eaten, and acids therefore absorbed, the stools are large, soft and readily evacuated. It is therefore easy to understand why fibre-rich food protects against constipation, piles and irritable bowels, and more serious conditions such as varicose veins, rupture of the gut (diverticular disease) and cancer. These are all caused by pressure, irritation and toxins in the lower gut.

Sir Richard Doll, Emeritus Professor of Medicine at Oxford University, is one of the men who established the link between cigarette smoking and cancer by epidemiological means. His investigation of the incidence of smoking and of cancer in different populations was of the same type as Dr Cleave's and Dr Trowell's studies of the link between refined carbohydrates and Western diseases. Sir Richard's view is that 80 to 90 per cent of cancers in Britain and America are preventable. And of the various causes of cancer—smoking, pollution, diet—he believes that diet plays a major, if not the major, role in cancer. In a BBC Radio 4 programme, speaking cautiously as scientists do, he said:

> There's quite strong, while far from conclusive evidence, that increasing the amount of cereal fibre in the diet will reduce the risk of cancer of the large bowel. It will certainly relieve constipation. It may help reduce the risk of diabetes. It may help reduce the risk of other so-called 'diseases of civilisation'.

On another occasion, in a preface to one of J L Cleave's books, Sir Richard wrote that if only a small part of Cleave's views proved true then he 'will have made a bigger contribution to medicine than most university departments or medical research units make in the course of a generation'. Sir Francis Avery Jones, the distinguished gastroenterologist, has gone further, saying that the work of Cleave and his supporters 'will prove to be, after antibiotics, the most important medical advance of this century'.

With this support, and with the publicity given to fibre by Audrey Eyton's *F-Plan Diet*, there is a danger that dietary fibre will gain the status almost of a medicine. As with vitamins, it would be a great pity if fibre were perceived as a supplement, to be eaten on top of unhealthy food from which fibre—and vitamins—has been processed.

It is certainly true that, in itself, fibre is necessary to health. It is also true that fibre-rich food is liable to be more satisfying than processed food. One study has shown that wholemeal bread is more satisfying than white bread. Given the choice and asked to eat until they felt comfortably full, ten out of twelve people ate less wholemeal bread than white bread; including the energy value of the butter, those who ate the wholemeal bread consumed 665 calories on average, those who ate white bread 825.

The food Audrey Eyton recommends in the *F-Plan Diet* is, together with that recommended by nutritionist Nathan Pritikin in his diet and exercise programmes, more healthy than any other diet regimes. But it is essential that the fibre-rich food is fresh and includes vegetables and fruit, along with wholewheat bread. From the health point of view some of Mrs Eyton's recommendations are not of great value: baked beans, for example, are high in fibre but, besides being processed and therefore robbed of nutrients, contain over 5 per cent refined sugar. Likewise, All-Bran, although a whole cereal, contains no less than 15.4 per cent refined sugar. While having less fibre than All-Bran, puffed wheat and shredded wheat are none the less very fibrous and contain very little refined sugar; eaten with fruit, they are healthier than All-Bran. Best of all is the sugar-free muesli that can be bought cheaply in bulk in most health food shops.

It is a pity that Mrs Eyton's recipes do not avoid refined sugar rather more explicitly. Like other diet books, the chief fault of her recommendations is that her regimes, of 1000 to 1500 calories a day, cannot contain enough nourishment. But anyone who cheats on the F-Plan and eats half as much again to twice the amount of food stipulated, and at the same time takes plenty of the type of exercise recommended in the next chapter of this book, will gradually and reliably lose fat and gain in health.

No single group of foods can supply all the nourishment we need. And fibre itself is a necessary package for nutrients rather than being a food in the sense of supplying energy or nourishment. Nevertheless it is true that we in the West should now think again about the food we eat and systematically shift our eating habits in favour of unprocessed carbohydrates. It is certain that if we do so, many 'Western' diseases will cease to be mass killers. It would be pleasant if people were to take individual responsibility for their own well-being, and put into effect the recommendations of the group of British doctors who have identified the crucial role of whole food in health and illness during the lifetime of those doctors.

### The poor eat grain

In 1973 the Food and Agricultural Organisation (FAO) and the World Health Organisation (WHO) jointly published the results of a massive survey by Dr J Périssé, an FAO expert, into eating habits in 85 countries. In the light of the discoveries by Cleave, Burkitt, Trowell and the other doctors, the results of the FAO survey have become a key to our new understanding of what is healthy food.

The survey divided the 85 countries into four groups. The countries with least money, with 760 million inhabitants, had an average income per head per year of less than $100. The countries with most money, including the Western nations, had an income of $600 to $2600 per head per year. The two intermediate groups of countries, with 605 million inhabitants between them, had an average income of $100 to $600 per head per year.

With a few exceptions the eating habits of the poorest countries proved to be profoundly different from those of the richest. And the change from a poor, or peasant, pattern of eating to a rich, or Western, pattern proved to be systematic, so that the habits of the intermediate groups of countries were more, or less, like those of the poor or rich countries, depending on the income earned per head in that country.

If food is categorised as protein, fat and carbohydrate—the conventional division—then the differences between the poor and the rich countries are remarkable enough. Measured as a percentage of total energy intake, protein consumption in the poor and rich countries was much the same: about 11 to 12 per cent. Fat consumption was massively different: 12 per cent in the poor countries rising to 40 per cent in the rich countries (such as Great Britain and the USA). Carbohydrate consumption dropped correspondingly, from about 77 per cent in the poor countries to 48 per cent in the rich. (By the time of the McGovern report on dietary goals for the USA in 1977, total carbohydrate consumption was estimated at 46 per cent and fat consumption at 42 per cent of total energy intake in North America. The figures for Great Britain today are not much different.)

But these figures disguise the really massive difference in eating habits. Since the invention of agriculture about 10,000 years ago, cereals, rich in starch and fibre and other nutrients, have been the staple food of mankind. All countries developed a staple grain with which to make bread or an equivalent food: wheat in Europe and North America, corn in South America; rice in the East; and millet, rye, barley and oats elsewhere. Contrary to Professor Yudkin's thesis, there is evidence from examination of fossil human teeth that pre-agricultural man was also a plant-eater and that carbohydrates in some form have always been a staple food.

The cultivation of wheat from a hybrid of wild wheat and goat grass encouraged human settlement and, with it, the cultivation of other starchy foods: the pea and bean family (also known as pulses and legumes) and root vegetables (including tubers; notably, in recent times, the potato).

Naturally enough, therefore, the FAO survey showed that the poor nations consume about 70 per cent of their energy from unrefined carbohydrate foods: cereals, and also pulses, legumes and root vegetables. These they eat lightly cooked or uncooked.

And almost all the protein and fat eaten comes from these foods, as vegetable protein and vegetable fat. Only a tiny percentage of energy comes from animal protein and fat—about 7 per cent in the poorest countries. The percentage of vegetable protein and fat amounts to about 16 per cent. The remaining 7 per cent is processed carbohydrate—mostly refined sugar. The main difference between these figures, researched in the early 1970s, and now is that consumption of refined sugar, which is distributed and sold cheaply all over the world nowadays, is steadily rising.

The poorest countries live at and below subsistence level. But at a more developed and fortunate level, a peasant, whose wealth is his land and his produce, may neither need nor use very much money, especially in a country of peasants: a peasant economy is largely one of barter. The food peasants eat they mostly grow themselves. In good times and on good land, this food, almost entirely produce from cereals and vegetables, will be plentiful and fresh.

Western countries, the richest countries, have moved from a peasant economy to one dependent on industrialisation, among the consequences of which is processed food. Food is processed not for reasons of health, but for reasons of trade. The food that makes money for industry is food that keeps and travels well; and of all such foods refined sugar is the chief. Having no life, refined sugar does not rot.

At the same time, the rich countries have the money to grow prodigious quantities of grain. Michel Cépède, a French professor who works for the FAO, has calculated that whereas an inhabitant of the Third World eats somewhat over 400 pounds of cereal a year, British and North American people consume five times as much—nearly a ton of cereal a year—almost all of which is fed to animals raised for food. The amount of cereal actually eaten in Great Britain, North America and other Western countries is not much more than one-third of the amount in the Third World. Only rich countries can afford to breed animals for meat.

Industrialisation brings with it reliance on processed food. In the nineteenth century the people who suffered most from processed food were the working classes in Western cities. Later, malnutrition from processed food spread to other parts of the world, for example to Asians who contracted beri-beri from eating processed, white rice while having no money with which to buy other nutritious food. The least fortunate people in Third World countries are now being converted from peasant economies by the spread of industrialisation; they can only afford processed food. Economic colonialism is sometimes grimly termed 'Coca-colonisation'.

### The rich eat sugar and fat

Western nations balance their protein, fat and carbohydrate by eating meat and animal products, which they can afford. The FAO figures show just how dramatically different Western food is from that of peasant countries. In the richest countries energy taken from animal protein is about 8 per cent of the whole; from animal fat (including dairy produce) about 30 per cent. The total of vegetable protein and fat consumed in the West is about 16 per cent. The colossal difference between the poor and the rich countries is in carbohydrates: the West eats less than one-third the amount of whole carbohydrate eaten in peasant countries, and this tends to be in the form of vegetables rather than cereals. As a result, the volume of cereal fibre (which provides greater protection against diseases of the gut) eaten in Western countries may be only one-fifth that eaten in peasant countries.

In the rich countries, industrialisation has replaced cereals as a staple food with processed foods, meat and dairy produce. Poor countries affected by industrialisation get the processed food without the meat and dairy produce. Ironically it is the peasant countries with the lowest income per head, where very little processed food is eaten, that give us some guide to the food we need to keep and gain our health. This table shows the contrast between the types of food eaten in peasant and in Western countries:

|  | *Energy consumed (%)* | |
| --- | --- | --- |
|  | Peasant | Western |
| Vegetable protein | 7 | 4 |
| Animal protein | 4 | 8 |
| *Total* | *11* | *12* |
| Vegetable fat | 9 | 10 |
| Animal fat | 3 | 30 |
| *Total* | *12* | *40* |
| Whole carbohydrate | 70 | 22 |
| Processed carbohydrate[1] | 7 | 26 |
| *Total* | *77* | *48* |
| Total vegetable foods | 93 | 62 |
| Total animal foods | 7 | 38 |

[1] including refined sugar

The conventional division of food is between protein, fat and carbohydrate, with energy value included. This is because these were the first divisions made by food chemists. Later, during this century, vitamins were identified and the value of vitamins and minerals established. So we are taught to think of foods as divided somewhat like a book, into a first part (energy—calories), a second part with three sections (protein, fat and carbohydrate) and then a lot of appendices with odd titles that tend to be skipped (vitamins, minerals). Unless we make a conscious decision not to do so, we are bound to think of food in this way simply because this is how books on nutrition are arranged.

Nutritionists and diet doctors, and their readers, are now accustomed to a dialogue (a monologue in the case of dieters, who are expected to keep quiet and obey) in which calories are regarded with suspicion; protein is praised; carbohydrates are condemned (usually); fat is condemned (almost always); vitamins are praised and touted (as a form of medicine); and, now, fibre is praised (also as a form of medicine—but where does it fit with the other categories?). No wonder many dieters are confused.

It is time to forget these divisions. Recent attempts to preserve the terminology by subdivisions (into polysaturated fat and polyunsaturated fat, for example; and simple and complex carbohydrates; not to mention monosaccharides, disaccharides, and polysaccharides) merely create a jungle of jargon. And the classification of foods rich in starch as 'carbohydrate', the confusion of starch with sugar, and the refusal to distinguish whole from processed foods (so that wholemeal bread is bracketed with refined sugar as 'carbohydrate' and is commonly believed to have no more value as food) is a series of mistakes, encouraged by food processors, that has damaged the civilian population of the West in this century more than any war.

The important divisions of food were well known in the West before this century. They are between vegetable and animal food; whole and processed food; and fresh and stale food. We eat animal food for taste, processed food for convenience, but we do not need them. Wholewheat bread, legumes and root vegetables, well prepared and eaten fresh and lightly cooked, are rich in starch. But their classification as 'carbohydrates' is arbitrary. The carbohydrate in them supplies energy to the body in a natural way, without causing the disturbances that result from eating refined sugar. But foods rich in starch are also rich in other nutrients. In different proportions, they also contain protein, fat, fibre, vitamins and minerals.

It is not necessary to be a vegetarian to be healthy. But it is necessary to re-think the relationship between animal and vegetable foods. 'Meat and two veg' is the wrong balance. The chief ingredients in a meal should be cereal or vegetable: so that, for example, the Italian staples of spaghetti and other pastas with olive oil, flavoured in different combinations with vegetables or herbs or cheese or meat, is good food (and better still if the pasta is wholewheat). Meat and dairy produce, now a staple in the West, should merely accompany cereals and vegetables or at the least should be eaten only occasionally. And while animal food eaten sparingly is of course nutritious, processed and stale food is always inferior to whole and fresh food.

All whole grains—wheat, corn, rice, millet, rye, oats—contain protein. So do the legumes—peas, beans, lentils. And so do tubers—potatoes, for example. Many dried beans have as high a protein content as meat; and nuts and seeds are rich in protein and also vegetable fat. We think of meat as protein and therefore as good for us, but much of the meat we eat could almost as well be classified as fat, rather than protein. Even if it has no visible fat, the flesh of meat from animals that are reared in cages and get no exercise, is shot through with fat; and animal fat is certainly implicated in heart disease.

Overleaf is a comparison from the standard textbook, *The Composition of Foods*, of the nutritive quality of five common foods commonly lumped together as 'carbohydrates': potatoes (fresh, baked in their skins); a whole cereal (wholewheat bread), compared with a processed cereal (white bread); a legume (lentils); and refined sugar. The measurements are percentages; the energy content is per 100 grams. The figures in bold type show that the food is an important source of the particular nutrient.

Unlike fibre, starch is nourishing: it supplies energy to the body and brain. But like fibre, the special quality of starch in its natural form is that it acts as a package for other nutrients—protein, fat, natural sugar, vitamins and minerals. The processing of food means that food can be preserved, and can travel and be stored for long periods of time. But processing is at the expense of nourishment.

Compare the foods in the table. Potatoes are an important source of vitamin C (much less so if they are old or peeled) and of three minerals, notably potassium, in which many people are deficient. Wholewheat bread is an important source of no less than fifteen vitamins and minerals, white bread of half this number—and some minerals are added to white bread in an attempt to make it more nutritious.

Like bread, lentils are an important source of protein and also of thiamine, or vitamin B1, lost in the processing of many foods. In utter contrast to the whole foods listed, refined sugar, processed more thoroughly than anything else we eat, is empty of nourishment.

When nutrition experts say, as they so often do in newspapers and magazines, that we get all the nourishment we need from a normal, balanced and varied combination of foods, they are in

|  |  | Potatoes | Bread (whole-wheat) | Bread (white) | Lentils | Sugar (refined) |
|---|---|---|---|---|---|---|
| Water | % | 71.0 | 40.0 | 39.0 | 72.1 | tr |
| Protein | % | 2.6 | **8.8** | **7.8** | **7.6** | tr |
| Fat | % | 0.1 | 2.7 | 1.7 | 0.5 | 0 |
| Starch[1] | % | **24.4** | **39.7** | **47.9** | **16.2** | 0 |
| Sugar[1] | % | 0.6 | 2.0 | 2.0 | 0.8 | **105**[2] |
| Fibre | % | **2.5** | 8.5 | **2.7** | **3.7** | 0 |
| Energy | cals | 105 | 216 | 233 | 99 | 394 |

*Vitamins*:

|  |  | Potatoes | Bread (whole-wheat) | Bread (white) | Lentils | Sugar (refined) |
|---|---|---|---|---|---|---|
| A (Carotene) | μg | tr | 0 | 0 | **60.0** | 0 |
| Thiamine (B1) | mg | 0.1 | **0.26** | **0.18** | **0.5** | 0 |
| Riboflavin (B2) | mg | 0.04 | **0.1** | 0.03 | **0.2** | 0 |
| Niacin (B3) | mg | 1.2 | **3.9** | 1.4 | 2.0 | 0 |
| Pyridoxine (B6) | mg | **0.2** | 0.14 | 0.04 | 0.11 | 0 |
| B12 | μg | 0 | 0 | 0 | 0 | 0 |
| Folic Acid (B) | μg | 10.0 | **39.0** | 27.0 | 5.0 | 0 |
| Pantothenic acid | mg | 0.2 | **0.6** | 0.3 | 0.3 | 0 |
| C (Ascorbic acid) | mg | **30.0** | 0 | 0 | tr | 0 |
| D | μg | 0 | 0 | 0 | 0 | 0 |
| E | mg | 0.1 | 0.2 | tr | 0 | 0 |
| Biotin (H) | μg | tr | **6.0** | 1.0 | 0 | 0 |

*Minerals*:

|  |  | Potatoes | Bread (whole-wheat) | Bread (white) | Lentils | Sugar (refined) |
|---|---|---|---|---|---|---|
| Sodium | mg | 8.0 | **540.0** | **540.0** | 12.0 | tr |
| Potassium | mg | **680.0** | 220.0 | 100.0 | **210.0** | 2.0 |
| Calcium | mg | 9.0 | 23.0 | **100.0** | 13.0 | 2.0 |
| Magnesium | mg | **29.0** | **93.0** | 26.0 | **25.0** | tr |
| Phosphorus | mg | 48.0 | **230.0** | 97.0 | **77.0** | tr |
| Iron | mg | 0.8 | **2.5** | **1.7** | **2.4** | tr |
| Copper | mg | **0.2** | **0.3** | 0.1 | **0.2** | 0.02 |
| Zinc | mg | 0.3 | **2.0** | 0.8 | **1.0** | 0 |
| Sulphur | mg | 42.0 | **81.0** | **79.0** | 39.0 | tr |
| Chloride | mg | 94.0 | **860.0** | **890.0** | 20.0 | tr |

[1] starch and sugar together are carbohydrate
[2] refined sugar contains what are in effect super-sweet elements
tr = trace

one sense correct. But in a more important sense they are misleading. The fact is that, compared with the food eaten at any other time in history, the food we in the West have eaten for the last six generations is uniquely abnormal, unbalanced and artificially varied. The cuisine food based on meat, dairy produce, refined sugar and processed flour developed by the middle classes in Western Europe in the eighteenth century as one means of boasting of their riches is still considered good food in Great Britain, the USA, France and other Western countries. But cuisine food is a source of sclerotic energy and has contributed to the premature death of countless hundreds of thousands of people. It represents the revenge of the black slaves on the descendants of their masters, who gorged themselves on the profits of the sugar trade.

### Fresh food—and fresh air

The table accompanying this chapter, 'The Staff of Life' (see page 140) is a guide to peasant food—the healthy food that has been the staple food of people throughout history. The principles of healthy food are easily set out.

Cereals, legumes and tubers, rich in starch and fibre and containing protein, fat, vitamins and minerals, are the natural staple foods of mankind. Of all these foods, wholewheat bread is the single most valuable food that is also a natural staple in the West.

Vegetables and fruit, containing starch or sugar and also vitamins and minerals, are a valuable complement to cereals, legumes and tubers, providing that they are eaten whole and fresh, and raw or undercooked.

Vegetable protein and fat are always a better source of nourishment than animal protein and fat, including dairy products. Nuts are a very valuable source of vegetable protein and fat, as are seeds.

Fresh food is always better than processed food. The closer food is to the earth the better. Vegetables are close to the earth;

meat further away; meat from animals that eat meat, such as pigs, further away still.

The recommendations made by the McGovern Senate Committee in 1977 and by the Royal College of Physicians in 1983 are a leap in the right direction. Both bodies had to deal with representations from the food and agriculture industries in the USA and Great Britain, however, and do not go far enough; their recommendations are in effect for important progress, not for an ideal. Given the availability and attraction of meat and dairy produce, but given also the need for health, a balanced distribution of food and a practical target at which everyone in the West could aim is as follows. (The current figures for the West and for peasant countries, and the McGovern/RCP recommendations, are given for comparisons.)

| | Peasant % | Western: % | McG/RCP % | Target % |
|---|---|---|---|---|
| Vegetable protein | 7 | 4 | - | 6 |
| Animal protein | 4 | 8 | - | 6 |
| *Total* | *11* | *12* | *12* | *12* |
| Vegetable fat | 9 | 10 | - | 12 |
| Animal fat | 3 | 30 | - | 12 |
| *Total* | *12* | *40* | *30* | *24* |
| Whole carbohydrate[1] | 70 | 22 | 48[2] | 60 |
| Processed carbohydrate | 7 | 26 | 10[2] | 4 |
| *Total* | *77* | *48* | *58* | *64* |
| Total vegetable foods | 93 | 62 | 70[2] | 82 |
| Total animal foods | 7 | 38 | 30[2] | 18 |

[1] starch and sugar
[2] estimates

In practice, 4 per cent processed carbohydrate will be difficult to achieve, because it depends on a meticulous elimination of processed food, sugar in particular. As things are in Great Britain now, this requires access to health food shops, plentiful in most cities but not in the countryside where so often, ironically, fresh unprocessed food is hard to come by. But these guidelines are a means of bringing back in balance the foods we eat.

The sure sign that food has been drained of nourishment is the increase in overweight and obesity. The worse the food, the fatter people get, for this is the only way they can get enough nourishment. And the increase in obesity and of diseases of the alimentary tract and the cardiovascular system are all inter-connected.

In the first chapter of this book I quoted a bewildered passage from one of Dr Robert Atkins' diet books in which he says that, if all else fails, a trip to the Mediterranean is recommended. It 'always seems to help with weight reduction. It may be something in the soil.' And I mentioned my month's holiday in Greece, during which I lost 8 pounds. Well, there is no cuisine food in Greece. Greek food remains peasant food, and authentic Greek food is the healthiest in Europe. During my long stay I got as close to the guidelines to healthy food outlined above, as I ever had in my life. Dr Atkins' shot in the dark finds a target.

What I also enjoyed in Greece that summer was plenty of fresh air. And for everybody who wants to lose fat while eating plenty of good food, the recipe is: peasant food, and more air.

## Table 2. The Staff of Life

Cereals, legumes, tubers, together with other vegetables, fruit, nuts, and seeds, have been the staff of life of all people throughout the world at all time of human history. Meat and dairy products are also enjoyed by hunter-gatherers, pastoralists, and peasants, but only on occasion and as accompaniments to the staple plant and vegetable foods. (There are two exceptions to this rule: Eskimo and Masai people.)

In the last 100-150 years, machines and money have together created a catastrophic aberration in the West. Rich people have made animal foods a staple; poor people have had to eat processed food. Most people now eat a combination of animal foods and processed foods. These are the prime cause of 'Western diseases' and also of overweight and obesity.

There are no recipes or instructions in this book. Instead, what follows overleaf is a guide to fifty foods available in Britain and America which, if taken as staple foods, and eaten in appropriate combination, are a good approximation to the peasant food that gives health, prevents disease, and, together with exercise, is proof against overweight and obesity.

Guidelines can be only of general use. Any reader wanting individual guidance to good food should write to me, Geoffrey Cannon, The Nutrition Association, 6 Aldridge Road Villas, London W11 1BP. Please mark your envelope 'Dieting Makes You Fat' and enclose a stamped addressed envelope.

Key

| *Vitamins* | | *Minerals* | |
|---|---|---|---|
| A | Carotene | S | Sodium |
| B1 | Thiamine | P | Potassium |
| B2 | Riboflavin | Ca | Calcium |
| Ni | Niacin (B3) | M | Magnesium |
| B6 | Pyridoxine | Ps | Phosphorus |
| Fo | Folic Acid (B complex) | I | Iron |
| Pa | Pantothenic Acid | Cu | Copper |
| C | Ascorbic Acid | Z | Zinc |
| E | | Su | Sulphur |
| Bi | Biotin (vitamin H) | Cl | Chloride |

| per 100 g | Water % | Protein % | Fat % | Starch % | Sugar % | Dietary Fibre % | Energy cals | Vitamins Good sources of | Minerals Good sources of |
|---|---|---|---|---|---|---|---|---|---|
| *Cereals* | | | | | | | | | |
| Bran, wheat | 8.3 | 14.1 | 5.5 | 23.0 | 3.8 | 44.0 | 206 | B1 B2 Ni Fo Pa | P Ca M I Z Cu Z |
| Bread, wholemeal | 40.0 | 8.8 | 2.7 | 39.7 | 2.1 | 8.5 | 216 | B1 B2 Ni Fo Pa Bi | S P M Ps I Ps Cu Z Su Cl |
| Crispbread, rye | 64.0 | 9.4 | 2.1 | 67.4 | 3.2 | 11.7 | 321 | B6 Fo Bi | S P M I Z |
| Flour, wholemeal | 14.0 | 13.2 | 2.0 | 63.5 | 2.3 | 9.6 | 318 | B1 B2 Ni B6 Fo Pa | S P M I Ps Cu Z Su Cl |
| Muesli | 8.6 | 13.2 | 7.5 | 47.8 | 3.9 | 19.0 | 388 | B2 Ni B6 E | S P M I Z |
| Oatcakes | 55.0 | 10.0 | 18.3 | 59.9 | 3.1 | 4.0 | 441 | B6 Fo E | S P M I Z |
| Puffed wheat | 2.5 | 14.2 | 1.3 | 67.0 | 1.5 | 15.4 | 325 | Ni B6 Fo E | P M I Z |
| Shredded wheat | 7.6 | 10.6 | 3.0 | 67.5 | 0.4 | 12.3 | 324 | Ni B6 Fo E | P I Z |
| Weetabix | 3.8 | 11.4 | 3.4 | 66.5 | 6.1 | 12.7 | 340 | B1 B2 Ni B6 Fo E | S P M I Z |
| *Legumes, etc.* | | | | | | | | | |
| Beans: | | | | | | | | | |
| broad (boiled) | 83.7 | 4.1 | 0.6 | 6.5 | 0.6 | 4.2 | 48 | A Pa | P Ps |
| haricot (boiled) | 69.6 | 6.6 | 0.5 | 15.8 | 0.8 | 7.4 | 93 | Fo | P Ps I Z |
| baked (in tomato sauce) | 73.6 | 5.1 | 0.5 | 5.1 | 5.2 | 7.3 | 64 | A Fo | S P M Su Cl |
| Lentils | 72.1 | 7.6 | 0.5 | 16.2 | 0.8 | 3.7 | 99 | A B1 B2 | P M Ps I |
| Peas, fresh (boiled) | 80.0 | 5.4 | 0.4 | 5.9 | 1.8 | 5.2 | 52 | B6 Fo | Cu Z |
| Sweetcorn | 65.1 | 4.1 | 2.3 | 21.1 | 1.7 | 4.7 | 123 | B6 Fo | S P M |
| Tomatoes | 93.4 | 0.9 | Tr | 11.0 | 9.1 | 2.3 | 14 | A Bi C E | P |
| *Root vegetables, tubers* | | | | | | | | | |
| Carrots (boiled) | 91.5 | 0.6 | Tr | 0.1 | 4.2 | 3.1 | 19 | A C | P |
| Parsnips | 83.2 | 1.3 | Tr | 10.8 | 2.7 | 2.5 | 56 | Fo C E | P |
| Potatoes, new (boiled) | 78.8 | 1.6 | 0.1 | 17.6 | 0.7 | 2.0 | 76 | B6 C | P M Cu |
| Potatoes, old (boiled) | 80.5 | 2.1 | 0.1 | 19.3 | 0.4 | 1.0 | 87 | B6 C | P M Cu |
| Potatoes (baked in jackets) | 57.5 | 2.1 | 0.1 | 19.8 | 0.5 | 2.0 | 85 | C | P |
| Turnips, boiled | 94.5 | 0.7 | 0.3 | 0 | 2.3 | 2.2 | 14 | Fo | P |
| *Leaf vegetables* | | | | | | | | | |
| Broccoli tops | 89.9 | 1.8 | Tr | 0.1 | 1.5 | 4.1 | 18 | A B2 B6 C E | P |
| Brussels sprouts | 91.5 | 2.8 | Tr | 0.1 | 1.6 | 2.9 | 18 | A B6 C | P |

| Food | | | | | | | | Vitamins (good sources) | Minerals (good sources) |
|---|---|---|---|---|---|---|---|---|---|
| Cabbage (boiled) | 95.7 | 1.3 | Tr | Tr | 1.1 | 2.5 | 9 | A B6 Fo C E | P Ca |
| Lettuce | 95.9 | 1.0 | Tr | 0.4 | 1.2 | 1.5 | 12 | A Fo C | P Ps |
| Spinach | 85.1 | 5.1 | 0.2 | 0.5 | 1.2 | 6.3 | 30 | A B2 Fo C E | P Ca M I |
| *Fruit* | | | | | | | | | |
| Apples | 64.9 | 0.2 | Tr | 0.1 | 9.1 | 1.5 | 35 | | P |
| Apricots | 86.6 | 0.6 | Tr | 0 | 6.7 | 2.1 | 28 | A | P |
| Bananas | 70.7 | 1.1 | 0.3 | 3.0 | 16.2 | 3.4 | 79 | A | P M |
| Blackberries | 82.0 | 1.3 | Tr | 0 | 6.2 | 7.3 | 29 | C E | P |
| Currants, black | 77.4 | 0.9 | Tr | 0 | 6.6 | 8.7 | 28 | Bi C | P |
| Currants, red | 82.8 | 1.1 | Tr | 0 | 4.4 | 8.2 | 21 | Bi C | P |
| Damsons | 77.5 | 0.5 | Tr | 0 | 9.6 | 4.1 | 38 | A B1 Pa C E | S Ca I |
| Figs, green | 84.6 | 1.3 | Tr | 0 | 9.5 | 2.5 | 213 | B6 | P |
| Grapes, black | 65.2 | 0.5 | Tr | 0 | 13.0 | 0.3 | 51 | | P |
| Grapes, white | 79.3 | 0.6 | Tr | 0 | 16.1 | 0.9 | 63 | | P |
| Lemons | 85.2 | 0.8 | Tr | 0 | 3.2 | 5.2 | 15 | B6 Pa C | P Ca |
| Oranges | 86.1 | 0.8 | Tr | 0 | 8.5 | 2.0 | 35 | Fo C | P |
| Peaches | 86.2 | 0.6 | Tr | 0 | 9.1 | 1.4 | 37 | A Ni | P I |
| Prunes (stewed) | 60.5 | 1.3 | Tr | 0 | 20.4 | 8.1 | 82 | A | P |
| Raspberries | 83.2 | 0.9 | Tr | 0 | 5.6 | 7.4 | 25 | Bi C E | P M Ps |
| Sultanas | 18.3 | 1.8 | Tr | 0 | 64.7 | 7.0 | 250 | B1 B6 E | P |
| *Nuts* | | | | | | | | | |
| Almonds | 4.7 | 16.9 | 53.5 | 0 | 4.3 | 14.3 | 567 | B2 Ni B6 Fo E | P Ca M I Z |
| Brazil nuts | 8.5 | 12.0 | 61.5 | 2.4 | 1.7 | 9.0 | 619 | B1 B6 E | P Ca M Ps I Cu Z S |
| Chestnuts | 51.7 | 2.0 | 2.7 | 29.6 | 7.0 | 6.8 | 470 | B2 B6 Bi | P M |
| Coconut, fresh | 42.0 | 3.2 | 36.0 | 0 | 3.7 | 13.6 | 351 | B6 C Fo | S P I |
| Peanuts, fresh | 4.5 | 24.3 | 49.0 | 5.5 | 3.1 | 8.1 | 570 | B1 Ni B6 Fo Pa E | P M I Z |
| Peanut butter | 1.1 | 22.6 | 53.7 | 6.4 | 2.1 | 7.6 | 601 | B6 Fo Pa E | S P M I |
| Walnuts | 23.5 | 10.6 | 51.5 | 1.8 | 3.2 | 5.2 | 525 | B1 Ni Fo Pa E | P Ca M Ps I Z |

Two vitamins of which the foods in this table are not good sources, are vitamin B12 and vitamin D. B12 is in various fish; animal livers; and eggs. D is in milk and cod liver oil; also in sunlight.

Table compiled by Kathy Crilley. Chief source of information: *McCance and Widdowson's The Composition of Foods* edited by A A Paul and D A T Southgate (HMSO 1978).

CHAPTER FIVE

# *More Air! More Air!*

Nothing affects cheerfulness less than wealth and nothing more
than health. Let us seek to maintain cheerfulness. Without
appropriate daily exercise no-one can remain healthy, because
satisfactory completion of all living functions requires movement
of the parts concerned as well as of the whole. Aristotle was right
to say 'life is motion'.
SCHOPENHAUER
*Aphorisms on the Wisdom of Life*


The narrower and more limited our lives become, the more vitally
necessary people will find it to satisfy their longing for freedom in
the hazard of their athletic performance.
ROGER BANNISTER
*The First Four Minutes*


## *Oxygen: the vital fuel*

Wealth, power and fame have their rewards, but most people
who live well manage without them. Sooner or later we all find
out that the most valuable prize in life is not a rare external
object but a common inborn quality: our health.

We in the West have had a negative attitude towards health.
We spend the first part of our lives thinking nothing of it, and
the second part afraid of losing it. We have been preoccupied not
with good health but with ill-health; not with well-being but with
disease. An unorthodox but apt definition of 'technology' is 'a

means whereby we avoid experiencing our own lives'. Medical technology—the medicine of drugs and surgery where the money, power, newspaper headlines and Nobel Prizes are—discourages us from being responsible for our own health. A long-running BBC Television series has the revealing title *Your Life in Their Hands*. We have the same attitude to doctors and surgeons as the little child who cries out 'Mummy, take the pain away!'

We associate the entire concept of disease with what is in fact a single type of disease: infections, which, while they can largely be prevented by good sanitation, can also be checked or cured by modern medicine. We tend to think of disease as a visitation, as bad luck, as something for which we have no responsibility. We ignore deficiency diseases, caused by lack of nourishment from food, because we assume they do not exist in the West. And we fear the misnamed 'degenerative' diseases of the heart, lungs and blood vessels, and of the alimentary tract. In some way we imagine that these, too, are visitations, whereas they are properly named 'Western' diseases, because they are caused by the circumstances in which we live and by our own habits.

It was not always so. The awareness that our good health is our responsibility, a treasure to be protected, is contained in our language. The words 'salute' and 'salutation' derive from *salus*, the Latin word for 'health'. It also means 'safety'. The common French and Italian greetings—*Salut!* and *Salute!*—are wishes for good health and well-being. In this country, greetings are more muted. But on formal occasions, speakers will propose each others' health; and sometimes over drinks, if the occasion seems right, you may toast a friend with the words 'your good health'. The old knowledge is still there, although half-buried.

As with good health, so with the universal element in our environment: air. People who spend most of their time sitting or lying, especially town and city dwellers, pay no attention to air. After all, as well as being everywhere, it is invisible. Scientists look for new drugs as zealously as alchemists looked for gold. In both cases, the irony is that the most precious element is the most common. Without air we die within five minutes. People who lead active lives value air. But, even more than with good health, people who lead sedentary lives remember the value of air only in extremity. On the point of drowning, the swimmer has one thought in mind; likewise, the person hemmed in by street crowds. The cry is the same. 'More air! More air!'

Oxygen is that part of air which is vital to all the functions of the body. Just as fuel is burned in a flame of oxygen to provide energy in the form of heat, so oxygen transforms the fuel we eat—food—into all the types of energy that make up life itself; not of course literally in a flame, but by agents in the body that oxidise the food. The dictionary defines 'food' as 'what one takes into the system to maintain life and growth'. This is why the great nutritionist Sir Robert McCarrison wrote: 'Strictly speaking oxygen and water are to be regarded as foods, for of all the supplies on which the cells of the body are dependent they are the chief.'

Which comes first, then: food or oxygen? In one sense the question has no meaning, for we need both, just as a domestic fire has no being without both fuel and oxygen. While the body's fire of course produces no flame, it produces energy in all the forms the body needs. And just as a domestic fire may burn well and brightly with different amounts of fuel and with different draughts, so we can live and thrive at very different levels of energy balance, between the energy supplied by food and that by oxygen.

In a vital sense, though, oxygen comes first. The purpose of the new-born infant's first cry is to take air into its lungs. Most people in the West are in a double bind. Not only do they suffer from eating processed, unnatural foods. They also suffer because they do not take the exercise that was a natural part of life before the car was invented. The first move to be free from this bind is to take in more oxygen, by means of appropriate exercise. The issue with food is not quantity, but quality. But the issue with oxygen is one of quantity: almost all of us will thrive if we get more of it. And once we start to use more oxygen, remarkable things start to happen.

## The desire to be fit

In Spring 1982 I launched what became known as the *Fun Runner '82* project with *Running* magazine. Having started to jog in 1978, I had run my first marathon, in Paris in 1980, and started to write a column for *Running*. In 1981 I launched the *London 1982/50* project. The title was meant to convey the project's aim: to train fifty men and women for the second London marathon in 1982. The project worked; and so I and about a dozen of the *1982/50* participants decided to encourage a group of absolute beginners to train, not for a marathon, but to complete the *Sunday Times* National Fun Run five months later, in September 1982. This was *Fun Runner '82*.

We reckoned that the Hyde Park Fun Run, which is 2½ miles long, was an attainable goal. 'To qualify, you have to be an absolute beginner,' I wrote.

> I'm looking for people who have never kept fit on any regular basis. I shall be especially interested if you're overweight, or smoke, or have had any history of debilitating illness, or in general feel that you're in such bad shape that the Fun Run seems an Everest.

The applications poured in, from couples, from men, from women.

> We suddenly realised we were getting old and out of condition when we got a dog that needed a lot of exercise.

This was from a couple aged 28. An ex-smoker who was toying with the idea of becoming an ex-drinker wrote:

> After the excesses of Christmas I looked into the mirror and was horrified to see a flabby 5'11", 14 stone, balding local government officer. Two of these factors could not be reversed, but I decided to do something about my weight and fitness.

Most of the letters were from people who thought, correctly, that they were overweight. One mother said that her family loved swimming, but that she no longer went because she was ashamed of her size. Two other letters from women said:

> I am 28, and have progressively got less and less fit during the last five years. My energy output is very low as I have an office job that entails sitting down all day. The time has come when I would love to be fit again.

And, from a middle-aged mother:

> Is this the answer to the feeling that my waist is sinking into my hips, is this the self-discipline I have vaguely been feeling I need?

Most of the overweight people were women whose weight had increased to, and then beyond, 10 stone and who had discovered that dieting doesn't work. Some had been humiliated by the emphasis on competitive sport at school:

> I was overweight during my school years and pretty useless at sports, always being the one that the coach had to wait for after the cross-country.

Many recalled a lost energy. These letters were wistful, moving, sometimes resigned, a few despairing:

> I have for some time felt generally below par and lacking in energy—the lack of positive health—since I came to London from the countryside.

Eventually I received 130 applications. The first 84 were analysed: four were asthma sufferers, three from people with high blood pressure already diagnosed. One person had a heart murmur. Other conditions included a pulmonary embolism (recovered); slipped discs (two), back problems, bronchitis, hernia, curvature of the spine and epilepsy. One of the most touching letters said:

> Medically the last 18 months have been rotten. Head, leg and shoulder injuries and an unknown virus took it out of me spiritually

as well as physically. However, I feel much better now, except that I feel the strain of being very overweight.

Of the 84, 22 smoked, 23 had given up; 49 were definitely overweight; 38 had taken no exercise since school and 40 said they had exercised 'a bit'. Their ages ranged from 18 to 55, most people in their 30s and 40s. The average age was early to mid 30s.

Eventually 64 people were chosen to take part in *Fun Runner '82*. The fittest participant was, at 55, the oldest: John Routledge, a company director. The previous summer he had been given an executive check-up. He was a bit alarmed at his blood pressure, but was told that it was not unusual for his age. A couple of months later he had a massive heart attack and then clinically 'died'. Afterwards, in hospital, he remembered a conversation with a friend playing snooker; he had leaned over the table to play a ball and couldn't reach. 'Your undercarriage is in the way, John,' said his friend. Out of hospital John started to jog and eat fresh food. He had lost about 30 pounds and was doing 5-mile runs when I met him. His experience as a runner should have disqualified him from joining the project; but his experience of heart disease and his subsequent decision to save his own life would, I thought, be valuable.

Vic Burrowes, one of the applicants had written:

> If I am selected for your programme it could change my whole way of life. You said it might seem an Everest to some people. At the moment I would liken it to climbing the whole Himalayan range.

I was interested to see what would happen to Vic.

The participants in the project all agreed to undertake a series of tests during the five-month training programme, leading up to the goal of the *Sunday Times* National Fun Run. The physiological tests, based on the work of Professor Per-Olof Åstrand in Stockholm, were supervised by Ted Charlesworth and Kevin Sykes of the Human Performance Laboratory at Chester College and had already been used to test the fitness of the Cheshire fire service and police. They were carried out three times: at the start of the project, at the mid-point and at the end of the 21 weeks.

As well as measurements of height, weight and various parts of the body, the tests were of blood pressure; body fat percentage (inessential fat); lung capacity; heart rate; cardiorespiratory fitness (fitness of the heart and lungs); and, finally, 'fitness category'. Everybody wanted to know 'How Fit am I?' Fitness category was determined by measuring the fitness of the heart and lungs in terms of the body's capacity to use oxygen, and resulted in the following grades: 'excellent', 'good', 'average', 'below average', 'poor'. This grading was based on measurements of tens of thousands of people carried out in Dallas, Texas, by Dr Kenneth Cooper, founder of the Aerobics Institute.

I was also interested to know how far individuals' mood, attitudes and personality might change as a result of exercise and getting fit. So Dr Barrie Gunter, a research psychologist with special knowledge of sport, asked everyone to fill in a long questionnaire at the beginning and end of the project. This was the 'Cattell 16 Personality Factor' test, a standard method of measuring shifts in personality.

I myself devised a questionnaire for everyone to fill in at the mid-point of the project. This was designed to find out why people had joined *Fun Runner '82*; what they were getting out of it; and whether their eating and sleeping habits were changing. I also wanted to find out if people's moods changed as a result of exercise.

### Health tests

The physiological tests are usually called 'fitness tests'. I prefer the name 'health tests', for what they measure is the health and strength of the heart, lungs and blood vessels. They are not a health check of the whole body, but none the less they are important.

It seemed to me at the time, and with more force now, that tests of the sort supervised by Ted Charlesworth and Kevin Sykes, which take about 25 minutes to carry out and are suitable for any able-bodied person whatever their state of fitness, should be available as part of a general practitioner's routine examination, not just for private patients but as part of the National Health Service. The machinery is not expensive. In 1980, 172,243 men and women died of coronary heart disease in Britain. Current estimates are that 60 per cent of deaths from heart disease are preventable; my own belief is that heart disease could be almost as rare a cause of death in Great Britain now as it was 100 years ago.

Walter Elkan, Professor of Economics at Brunel University, estimates that the cost of heart disease in Britain was 26 million working days in 1979–80, at a total cost of perhaps £420 million. Professor Elkan estimates that the total cost of drugs to treat coronary heart disease is of the order of £215 million a year to the NHS. We still live in a world, though, where prevention, while cheaper than cure, is less glamorous, even when the immensely expensive 'cure' involving coronary by-pass, heart transplants and plastic hearts is unlikely to prove effective.

The initial series of physiological tests showed that on average the Fun Runners were a bit overweight and over-fat; that their blood pressure was marginally above the 'ideal' of 120/80 for women (at 127/91) and somewhat higher for men (at 137/93); and that fitness level was about 'average' for men and a bit 'below average' for women. 'Average' fitness is nothing to be satisfied about; it is what it says, the average for a basically sedentary population. The averages concealed a wide range of fitness. Of the 25 men assessed before they started to exercise, 6 were 'below average' and 2 'poor'. The women's fitness level was lower; of the 32 women measured, 5 were 'below average' and 10 'poor'. The 'poor' rating means you are liable to get out of breath running a bath.

The Fun Runners were formed into six teams, ideally each of ten to a dozen people. Experience shows that this is a good number for a team and allows for a few people to be away (on summer holiday, for instance). Each team had two trainers: these were mostly people from the now-completed *London 1982/50* project who had told me that they had gained so much from their nine months that they wanted to put back some of their enthusiasm, time and experience to the beginner Fun Runners.

Once a week every team met with their trainers. Once a month everybody came together on a Saturday morning in Hyde Park for a 'family' run. Special T-shirts were printed. Everybody was asked to exercise four times a week, preferably evenly spaced, and to keep a diary in which they recorded the times and distances they covered.

When starting an exercise programme, it is crucial to take it easy at first and then build up slowly. At first everybody was asked to jog and walk just over a mile, stopping whenever they liked. (Unfit people can usually run 200 to 400 yards without stopping.) As time went on everybody was encouraged to jog, and then run, further and faster, in their own time and at their own speed. The secret with this kind of training is to take your pulse rate and check to see that it is neither too high nor too low. (A guide to a training programme that able-bodied people can use is in the table 'Health Through Fitness', on pp. 183–6.)

At the mid-point of the project everybody had their second fitness tests. Allan Appleton, a 46-year-old company director, who had started the project with 'below average' fitness had risen to 'excellent'. In five months he was to lose 22 pounds in weight and 30 per cent of his non-essential body fat. But for him the main benefits at the half-way stage were:

> Many, and much appreciated: a tremendous increase in fitness and well-being, the previously unknown pleasure of running with members of my family. I will, for the rest of my life, run and exercise regularly.

You don't often hear people being this enthusiastic about a diet regime. Allan's loss of weight and non-essential fat was unusually high. I spent most time during the project with the 'Inner' team in central London, one of the six teams which included John

Routledge and Vic Burrowes. At the half-way stage, after eleven weeks, their results were:

|  | Age | Body weight (st:lb) | | Body fat (%) | | Fitness category | |
|---|---|---|---|---|---|---|---|
|  |  | before | after | before | after | before | after |
| Cinnia Bermingham | 36 | 9:1 | 8:9 | 16 | 14 | 5 | 2 |
| Victor Burrowes | 46 | 12:10 | 11:1 | 18 | 14 | 3 | 2 |
| Tim Burton | 31 | 11:7 | 11:11 | 15 | 14 | 4 | 3 |
| David Dyke | 34 | 10:5 | 10:0 | 19 | 15 | 4 | 1 |
| Nick Gray | 25 | 12:1 | 11:13 | 13 | 12 | 3 | 1 |
| Lynette Hadfield | 39 | 10:9 | 10:7 | 30 | 27 | 5 | 4 |
| Jane Heywood | 33 | 10:6 | 9:13 | 13 | 11 | 1 | 1 |
| Teresa Malinowska | 27 | 11:5 | 11:3 | 20 | 14 | 4 | 3 |
| Liz Parry | 29 | 11:0 | 10:11 | 22 | 20 | 5 | 3 |
| John Routledge | 55 | 11:11 | 11:9 | 11 | 10 | 2 | 2 |
| Eileen Ward | 27 | 15:1 | 15:5 | 40 | 38 | 5 | 4 |

Victor Burrowes had lost 23 pounds in eleven weeks. He had a sad tale to tell:

One of the reasons for taking up *Fun Runner '82* was excessive weight. Now, 11 weeks into the project I have lost almost two stone and my clothes still don't fit me! I shall have to buy a new wardrobe.

What's more, Vic swore that he had not been on a diet. Answering my questionnaire about food, he said that, while he was eating less sweets, he was eating more meat, fish, protein, fruit and vegetables. He also turned out to have a natural talent for running: he entered a 3-mile race and came second in the 46–50 age category. And he continued to enjoy his beer.

Tim Burton was the 14-stone local government officer who had written to me a few months before. Before starting to exercise he had gone on a semi-starvation diet, which he stopped as soon as he started to run. But having dieted he was weakened, and his fitness level at the start was the lowest of all the men. After eleven weeks he had gained over four pounds, but had lost body fat.

The most striking example of the way exercise affects body composition rather than weight was Teresa Malinowska, a tall young woman. She had lost a couple of pounds, and was to lose a total of 5 by the end of five months; but in eleven weeks she lost 30 per cent of her inessential body fat. Her body shape changed remarkably; as well as looking radiant, from being a bit plump she changed to being lean.

Jane Heywood started—and ended—the fittest in the group. She was in the habit of cycling to work. Eileen Ward was one of the three very over-fat women in the group of sixty-four, none of whom lost weight during the five months of the project, although all lost a small amount of fat. John Routledge showed no change in weight, body fat, or fitness, which was no surprise, because he was not taking any more exercise. At the beginning of the project his blood pressure, now much lower than the year before, was 144/86. In eleven weeks it came down to 120/80: the blood pressure of a young man.

### How to prolong your own life

While the project was running I heard a doctor say on BBC radio, without a doubt in his voice, that people with high blood pressure usually had to take drugs indefinitely to reduce the pressure. A leaflet put out by the Flora margarine project for heart disease prevention, found in many health centres, advocates losing weight, eating less salt, and cutting down saturated fats, together with giving up smoking and avoiding tension, as means to reduce blood pressure. No mention of exercise.

Yet in eleven weeks the blood pressure of all those participants who were measured twice fell as follows:

|  | before | after |
|---|---|---|
| Men | 137/93 | 127/82 |
| Women | 127/91 | 121/82 |

Dr Eoin O'Brien and Professor Kevin O'Malley explain the significance of these figures. They take the example of a man somewhat older than most men in *Fun Runner '82*:

A 45 year old man with a systolic pressure of 120 and a diastolic level of 80 may expect to live to over 70 years of age. A man of much the same age with a systolic presuure of 140 and a diastolic of 95 may expect to live six years less.

The fifteen people of the sixty-four who started the five-month projcet with high blood pressure ended with lower blood pressure. Here is the entire list:

|  |  | before | after |
|---|---|---|---|
| Women: | age 36 | 137/95 | 108/72 |
|  | 29 | 134/105 | 112/80 |
|  | 29 | 134/97 | 113/69 |
|  | 39 | 154/111 | 135/88 |
|  | 38 | 132/114 | 125/81 |
|  | 29 | 136/91 | 117/79 |
|  | 47 | 139/98 | 130/70 |
|  | 33 | 138/81 | 125/75 |
| Men: | age 46 | 152/106 | 130/74 |
|  | 31 | 146/91 | 140/86 |
|  | 53 | 158/108 | 130/90 |
|  | 25 | 142/90 | 135/78 |
|  | 55 | 144/86 | 120/80 |
|  | 48 | 140/90 | 125/66 |
|  | 26 | 140/80 | 122/63 |

In five months half a dozen people in their late 30s, 40s or 50s improved their life expectancy by six years. The man of 48 whose blood pressure dropped so remarkably was Rodney Lewis, a north London taxi-driver. Before the project, he said, he was always pushing his window down and shouting and screaming at silly drivers. His new blood pressure brought a new personality with it; he lost his jagged edges and became a calmer man. Vic Burrowes' blood pressure dropped more than 20 points.

Between May and September about ten people dropped out of the project; holidays and other reasons meant that others were not tested three times. Of those who completed the course (and the Fun Run) and were also tested in May, July and September, the men, on average, lost 9 pounds of body weight and, more significantly, over 20 per cent of their non-essential body fat. One man, Tim Burton, gained weight in the five months—all lean tissue. One stayed the same; two kept the same weight but lost fat; the rest lost weight and fat.

The women's results were less striking. On average they lost 4½ pounds of weight and 10 per cent of their non-essential fat. The three very over-fat women got fitter and completed the 2½-mile Fun Run to tumultuous cheers; but one did not change her weight or shape much, and the other two actually gained weight, while at the same time losing fat, over the five months. Paradoxically, they were the two who, at 14 stone 4 and 15 stone 1, had most to lose; both were also short in stature. Leaving these three women aside, the rest, half of whom were overweight, half average or slim, lost about 6 pounds in five months.

Losing weight was not, it should be said, a principal reason why people joined the project. In July, half-way through, I asked everybody why they had joined, and the most frequently mentioned reasons were 'getting fit', 'feeling good' and 'getting in shape'. Defined in this way, the project was a great success for almost everybody who completed it. This table compares the cardiorespiratory fitness of the 34 people who completed all the tests before and after the project.

|  | Men | | Women | |
|---|---|---|---|---|
|  | before | after | before | after |
| Excellent | 1 | 11 | 2 | 6 |
| Good | 2 | 3 | 4 | 8 |
| Average | 7 | 0 | 1 | 4 |
| Below average | 4 | 0 | 5 | 1 |
| Poor | 0 | 0 | 8 | 1 |

What impressed me equally were the comments people made about their eating habits. In July, half-way through, I asked participants how much they were eating, and if they had changed their food habits in any way. Everyone had been strongly advised to keep their strength up and not diet, and in July only one person said she was on a diet. If anything, people seemed to be eating more, not less.

I also asked if people were spontaneously eating more or less of different types of food. The only outside influence was Audrey Eyton's *F-Plan Diet*, advocating fibre, which became the thing to eat in the summer of 1982. Members of the project were asked to list the types of food they were eating more, or less, of:

| Foods | more | less |
|---|---|---|
| Meat/fish | 10 | 6 |
| Dairy products | 9 | 10 |
| Sugar/sweets/chocolate | 7 | 18 |
| Cereals and pastas | 12 | 7 |
| Fibre | 15 | 1 |
| Alcohol | 10 | 17 |
| Protein | 9 | 3 |
| Fat | 0 | 14 |
| Carbohydrate | 9 | 6 |
| Vitamins | 11 | 2 |
| Fruit | 21 | 2 |

The men and the women responded similarly. Replies to questionnaires of this sort must be treated with some caution. Everybody knows that it is a good thing to eat fruit and vegetables, and a bad thing to eat fat, and people no doubt tend to report what they know they ought to do rather than what they actually do. Given this, it was quite striking that ten people said they were drinking more alcohol (usually in the form of beer after runs, judging by the jovial occasions I attended).

The switch away from sugar, sweets and chocolate in favour of cereals and pastas was therefore especially interesting. Sugar and products heavy in sugar are advertised as sources of quick energy, and runners are often (wrongly) told to eat them after a run. By contrast cereals and pastas have a stodgy image, and people who want to lose weight are often (wrongly) told to avoid them. But the Fun Runners moved away from refined carbo-hydrates—sugar, and also products heavy in sugar and fat—and moved towards whole carbohydrates—starch, and foods rich in fibre and natural sugar.

After eleven weeks of their exercise programme, the Fun Runners were approximating to the recommendations of the Royal College of Physicians spontaneously, without any prompting from doctors, books, trainers, or from me. Indeed, the shift in their eating habits away from refined sugar and in favour of starch came as a surprise.

### How to eat as much as you like

The implications of these results are exciting. They suggest that when people become active their bodies tend to adapt, to prefer foods rich in nourishment that supply energy at a natural rate and to avoid foods poor in nourishment that supply energy at an unnaturally fast rate. To put it another way, the fit body becomes healthy partly by adapting to prefer healthy food. Moreover, one vitamin, thiamine (B1) is used particularly in activity; and many unprocessed starchy foods are rich in thiamine.

I mentioned these findings to a leading expert on diabetes; for it is now recognised that adult-onset diabetes can be treated by cutting out sugar and by eating food rich in starch and fibre. 'Ah,' he said. 'You're one of those people who believes in the wisdom of the body.' Yes, I said, I supposed that I was.

On 26 September the members of the project had the time of their lives, running in the *Sunday Times* National Fun Run. A lot of the men had become pretty fast: most of them completed the 2½-mile course in under 18 minutes, and Rodney Lewis beat me by a second (he was in the same race as me, but I never managed to catch him). The women were less competitive. Debbie Hoyle, a young mother of two children, finished in 18 minutes 26 seconds; and Cinnia Bermingham, who had written to me five months before saying that she got out of breath running for a bus, finished in 19.06. The biggest cheers were for the women in their late 30s and 40s, some of whom had developed a fair turn of speed.

After five months, the project had encouraged a lot of people to become fit. But very much more had happened, besides. People had lost weight, lost body fat and changed shape. Their blood pressure had come down to that of young people, and, correspondingly, their ability to use oxygen had increased dramatically. They had proved to their own satisfaction that runners are healthy people.

Dr Barrie Gunter made his own assessment of the project. He said that after 21 weeks of exercise the Fun Runners were more self-confident and emotionally stable, more self-assured, more relaxed and composed. He was especially interested in how friendly most people had become. He said:

> My feeling is that this is partly a result of taking part in a group activity with other people all striving towards the same goal; as well as training their bodies, people were also exercising their skills in dealing with other people. The less fit had been helped and encouraged by the more fit.

These benefits are part of what running is all about. Running is, almost uniquely, a social activity, because you can not only run with companions (as opposed to competing against an opponent) but also talk with your companions all the time you are running—well, at least until the run becomes a little competitive.

Bill East is 53. At the end of the project his blood pressure had dropped by more than twenty points. He said:

> I have achieved far more than I thought possible. I can run 4½ miles non-stop, my weight, blood pressure and resting heart-rate are all down, and without trying my smoking is down. And I have learned that the body does not deteriorate pro rata with age: I am not that far behind youngsters half my age.

I was surprised to discover Bill's age. He looks ten years younger. Will Chapman was one of the leaders of the *Fun Runner* project. In 1971, weighing 16½ stone, he had a heart attack.

Afterwards, like John Routledge, he started jogging and became a marathon runner. He said:

> Non-runners ask me what I get out of pounding the streets. My weight is a normal 12½ stone and yet I eat and drink what I want; I'm told I look young for my 45 years and I feel great.

Will was a member of the previous *London 1982/50* project, but there is no need to run marathons to benefit from exercise. Bobbie Randall is 47 and the mother of six. 'I'm the only fatty left in the family,' she explained, writing to join *Fun Runner '82*. 'My job is sedentary, as are my hobbies. I just cannot shift my surplus. Perhaps it's been around too long.' In five months she lost 11 pounds, her blood pressure was down from 139/98 to 130/70, her ability to use oxygen had almost doubled, and she ran the Fun Run in 23 minutes 50 seconds, coming 71st out of 141 in her age category. In January 1983 she won a 4.2-mile handicap race organised by the Serpentine Running Club. Rodney Lewis had been a previous winner of this race.

## Lose weight: eat more

I was already aware that Professor Peter Wood was mounting similar projects in California with a number of colleagues. Wood, an Englishman who has lived in the USA for twenty years, is deputy director of the Heart Disease Prevention Unit at Stanford University, and a veteran of over seventy marathon races. He is also jointly responsible for a nationwide club of veteran joggers and runners, the '50+ Association'.

In 1976 he mounted a 17-week exercise programme for twenty-two very overweight women aged between 30 and 52. Most had previously tried and failed to lose weight by dieting. The women also attended classes designed to encourage awareness of their eating habits, but were not told to diet. In practice, most of them made moderate reductions in the amount of food they ate.

At the end of the programme, average weight had fallen by 9

pounds. Body fat had decreased by 11 pounds, while lean tissue had increased by 2 pounds. Resting heart rate and heart rate recovery after exercise also decreased, as did blood pressure. Wood's professional speciality is the study of blood lipids; that is to say, fat in the blood. It is now known that the volume of fat in the blood does not itself indicate a high risk of heart disease. What matters is the type of fat. It is 'low density lipoprotein' (LDL), large, sticky globules of fat bound up with protein, that are linked with heart disease. LDL increases when large amounts of refined sugar are eaten, and in time the sticky globules line and clog the blood vessels. 'High density lipoprotein' (HDL) by contrast, small, smooth globules of fat and protein, is not only harmless but may in effect scour the blood vessels, renewing them and making them healthier.

Wood found that exercise increased the volume of HDL and decreased that of LDL, and also significantly increased the proportion of HDL to LDL. His findings have been confirmed by work done by Dr Peter Williams of BUPA, in London.

Wood's next projects were more ambitious. He compared the amount of food eaten by 34 male and 27 female runners aged between 35 and 59, and averaging 35 to 40 miles a week.

As might be expected, the runners were considerably leaner and lighter than the 'control' group. But the runners were eating more—a lot more.

Male runners consumed 2959 calories a day, vs 2361 for controls. The corresponding mean values for female runners and controls were 2386 and 1817 calories a day, respectively.

The runners were considerably lighter than the non-runners. The male runners were eating almost half as much again per pound of body weight as male non-runners; women more than half as much again. Lose weight: eat more. Gain weight: eat less. As the Royal College of Physicians' report said in 1983:

The role of physical activity in the development of increased adiposity may well have been under-emphasised. . . . There will need to be an appreciable and permanent change in society's attitude to exercise.

Not everybody wants to run 35 to 40 miles a week. And sedentary people often assume that the only way to lose weight and fat and become slim by running is either to have run all your life or else to run great distances. Another study by Peter Wood, of middle-aged women who played 10 hours of tennis a week, compared with a control group of sedentary women, disproves that. Wood: 'We found that the tennis players' food intake was close to 2400 calories a day, while the overweight women ate only 1400. That's an enormous difference.'

That is not to say that the runners and the tennis players studied were eating a great deal: but at 2400 to 3000 calories a day their energy intake was sufficient to ensure them enough nourishment from vitamins and minerals, given that the food eaten is nutritious. Rather, it was the inactive people who ate little; in the tennis study, the inactive women, who on average were overweight, consumed no more energy than many diet books recommend for a semi-starvation regime.

The full significance of this pioneering work becomes clear when the energy value of running and playing tennis is measured. Running uses about 9 to 12 calories a minute more than sitting, playing tennis about 5 calories more. Hence the estimate made by Dr John Garrow that running a marathon consumes about 2500 calories. Hence, also, the notion that you have to walk up and down Ben Nevis to work off the effects of a hearty meal.

The runners studied by Wood were eating 550 calories a day more than the non-runners. According to the usual calculations, in order to run that extra energy off, at a brisk 7 to 8 miles an hour, they would have to run for about an hour every day, or 50 to 65 miles a week—far more than they were actually running. Even a fast runner would have to do 45 miles a week to burn off 600 calories a day. Moreover, the runners were lighter than the non-runners.

The same calculation applied to the tennis players has even

more remarkable results. According to the books, you would have to play tennis for 200 minutes a day to burn off 1000 calories, which is 23 hours 20 minutes every week. In fact, the tennis-players were playing less than half that time. Something is missing from the calculations.

### Exercise speeds you up

In theory, according to the books, exercise is not a particularly effective way of losing weight and fat. In practice, according to experience, exercise can be a most effective way of losing some weight and more fat. Moreover, in Peter Wood's words:

> It is a fallacy that thinner, active people eat less than overweight, sedentary people. In fact, they eat more. We have proved that food intake increases among those who exercise and decreases among the sedentary.

Just as dieting slows you down, exercise, of the right type, speeds you up. What is missing from the calculations made of the energy cost of exercise is the fact that certain types of exercise, including running, speed up the metabolic rate, not only while you exercise but also afterwards.

As long ago as 1935 it was calculated that strenuous exercise such as football raises the resting metabolic rate by as much as 25 per cent for fifteen hours afterwards, and by about 10 per cent for forty-eight hours afterwards. Thus if you jog or run for ten minutes, you burn 90 to 120 calories more than you would at rest, and you continue to burn more for some time. The extent to which the resting metabolic rate remains higher after exercise varies with the individual and the type of exercise. A relatively heavy man uses half as many calories again in a run as a relatively light woman and will therefore burn more calories afterwards.

The facts that metabolism is dynamic, and that exercise using a lot of oxygen speeds up the metabolic rate and also improves health as well as fitness, are so important and basic that people often say to me: 'If all this is true, why haven't I heard it before?'

Fit and healthy people tend to be able to do without junk food and drugs; and junk food and drugs are very profitable commodities. That's one, cynical, reason. And preventative medicine remains the Cinderella of the medical profession, although that is now beginning to change. But there are a number of practical reasons why what is written here is likely to be news to many readers.

The procedure involved in measuring metabolic rate is complicated and laborious. Far more measurements have been made of changes in metabolic rate as a result of dieting, fasting and over-eating than as a result of exercise, simply because it is easier to measure people sitting down than to measure them running over a period of months.

Diet books and studies of obesity pay little attention to the role of oxygen because until recently the only group of people, mountaineers and divers aside, with a direct interest in the relationship of oxygen and energy balance were athletes. Exercise physiology, the science concerned with the effects of oxygen on the human body, was a specialised department, of general interest only to physical education teachers and trainers. Ordinary people took oxygen for granted, just as nutritionists who measure the energy content of food by burning it in a 'calorimeter' take it for granted.

But now the explosion of interest in exercise among ordinary citizens, and in particular the enthusiasm for jogging and running, is turning hundreds of thousands of previously fat people into athletes. These people find they no longer need to diet, and become interested in eating lots of good food instead. The scientists who study energy balance in fat people and those who study energy balance in fit people are beginning to get together.

The research now being done on exercise and metabolic rate is almost all new, and would have been hard to mount until recently for another practical reason. Research needs subjects. Until the late 1970s virtually everybody in Western countries remained sedentary throughout life, or else was active only when young. A few people remained active throughout life. For practical purposes it was unknown for people to get more active as they got older. Professor Jeremy Morris, whose studies of London bus conductors and drivers in the 1950s showed that because they walked up and down the stairs of the double-decker buses conductors were less likely to suffer heart disease, did his work at a time when doctors commonly believed that exercise was bad for you.

Conclusive studies of the effects of exercise on metabolism can only be carried out on people who, like the 64 Fun Runners, have decided for themselves to progress from being *homo sedentarius* to *homo sportivus*.

## The types of exercise

What is the effect of long-term, regular exercise on metabolic rate, on the quantity and quality of food eaten, on weight, shape, fitness and health? How much exercise is needed to become fit and healthy? Are some forms of exercise better than others? How long should exercise sessions take, and how regular should they be? It is only in the last few years that these questions could be answered with confidence.

In the remainder of this chapter I shall explain how any able-bodied person can get fit and healthy by means of exercise. The answers to the questions above are implied in two sentences in the Royal College of Physicians' report on obesity:

The physiological effects of short periods of moderately intensive exercise are well defined, and a minimum of 20 minutes of moderate activity three times a week seems sufficient to maintain cardio-vascular responses to physical activity. This degree of activity also seems to play an important role in improving an individual's sense of well-being.

That is to say, a certain type of exercise, carried out with a certain regularity for a certain amount of time, makes you feel good, makes you fit, and makes you healthy. The exercise that produces these effects is so-called 'aerobic' exercise.

Dr Kenneth Cooper is the founding father of the aerobic movement, first in the USA, and now throughout the world. In his book *Aerobics* he divides exercise into four types.

*Isometrics* tense the muscles against themselves or against an immovable object. Isometric exercises strengthen skeletal muscle and are useful for the bedridden and for astronauts. Sometimes they are recommended for executives and office workers who want to do battle with their desks.

*Isotonics* contract the muscles and also involve movement. As well as strengthening muscle they can make the body more supple or bulkier with muscle. They promote well-being as well as muscular fitness. Examples are the Canadian Air Force exercises in the popular book *Physical Fitness*, weight training, school PT and yoga.

*Anaerobic exercise* itself divides into two types: either too easy, or too hard, to be aerobic. Aerobic exercise requires a sustained supply of oxygen. Anaerobic exercise may be so gentle, or so brief, that it makes no real demands on the heart and the lungs. Alternatively, anaerobic exercise may be so intense that after a short while it cannot be sustained; the body cannot supply the volume of oxygen required and goes into 'oxygen debt', signalled by severe breathlessness.

*Aerobic exercise* occupies the middle ground between the two types of anaerobic exercise outlined above. It is neither gentle nor intense. It is exercise sustained at a steady, vigorous level for a considerable period of time.

Isometrics and isotonics do not increase the amount of oxygen used by the body, unless they are accompanied by systematic and sustained breathing exercises. Thus, they do not strengthen the heart, lungs and blood vessels and so improve fitness as distinct from health.

Any kind of sprinting, whether running, cycling or swimming, is by definition anaerobic, for sprinting cannot be sustained for more than a couple of minutes. 'Aerobics', now popular in Great Britain and the USA, is a mixture of dance and exercise which is aerobic simply because, properly taught, it is sustained for over five minutes at a time. What constitutes aerobic activity depends on the state of fitness and health of the individual. A gentle jog may be anaerobic for the fit young person because it is too easy; for the unfit middle-aged person it may be anaerobic because it is too hard.

Dr Cooper defines aerobic exercise for young people as follows:

> If the exercise is vigorous enough to produce a sustained heart rate of 150 beats a minute or more, the training-effect benefits begin about five minutes after the exercise starts and continue as long as the exercise is performed. If the exercise is not vigorous enough to produce or sustain a heart rate of 150 beats a minute, but is still demanding oxygen, the exercise must be continued considerably longer than five minutes, the total period of time depending on the oxygen consumed.

Fitness training may develop physical speed, strength or endurance in different proportions, depending on its purpose. This is true for the Olympic athlete, the patient recovering from a heart attack and for ordinary citizens, whatever their initial level of fitness.

The athlete trains in order to improve performance. A sprinter develops speed rather than endurance; a marathon runner develops endurance rather than strength. Training for many sports is specialist. And a fit person may or may not be a healthy person, depending on the type of training they undertake. Exercise that develops strength or speed but not endurance is anaerobic. Exercise that develops endurance is aerobic, because endurance is achieved by training the body's capacity to use oxygen. Aerobic exercise promotes health through fitness because, by its sustained use of oxygen, it strengthens the heart, lungs, blood vessels and other vital organs, as well as the muscles.

This is why, as Dr Cooper states, in order to be aerobic exercise must elevate the heart rate past a certain point for a certain period of time. The reason why sprinting is anaerobic is because it uses oxygen stored within the muscle itself, which is soon exhausted. On the other hand jogging (at a speed appropriate to the physical condition of the individual) is aerobic, because it uses oxygen breathed in from the air.

The key to aerobic exercise is that it should be sustained for five minutes at the very least, preferably for ten minutes; and that during this time the heart rate should be elevated to 60 to 80 per cent of its maximum. This duration and intensity has been determined by doctors and scientists specialising in the heart and in exercise physiology. Below the level of 60 per cent, exercise will not have an aerobic effect. And only very fit people can gain aerobic benefit from exercise above the 80 per cent level.

Some men (it's always men) push themselves too hard on exercise programmes, and there is even a condition known as 'positive addiction': the jogger cannot do without the daily session. I see no harm in running a lot if you enjoy it; but I always advise people, including runners training for marathons, to run no more than four days a week.

Progress in running and other aerobic activities is much like progress in any other area of life: it goes by fits and starts. You reach a certain level, then stick on this 'plateau' for a while, sometimes quite a long time; then there is a 'breakthrough' to a higher level. It's important not to expect progress to be steady. Many training programmes make that mistake.

These are the most common questions people ask me about aerobic exercise. First: which sports and activities are aerobic, and which are anaerobic? Second: how can I discover when my heart rate is elevated to 60 to 80 per cent of maximum? Third: how long should I exercise each day and each week? Fourth: how long will it take for the exercise to have a good effect on my health?

The 'Health Through Fitness' table on pages 183–6 is a guide to an aerobic exercise programme that any able-bodied person can follow and is designed to take the mystery out of aerobic exercise. It has been devised in consultation with Dr Cooper and Professor Peter Wood and also with Tom McNab (British athletics coach at the Munich and Montreal Olympics) and

Malcolm Emery (Head of Sports Sciences at the West London Institute).

If you can, join your local jogging club or aerobics group. If you have any doubts about your health, see your doctor and explain that you are about to take regular exercise. If your doctor thinks that exercise is unhealthy, insist on seeing a doctor who agrees with exercise. The advantage of joining a jogging club or aerobics class is that you should then have access not only to experienced people who can guide you but also to doctors expert in the treatment of fit and healthy people as opposed to ill people. Motivation is the special advantage of a club or group: everybody in the *Fun Runner '82* project agreed that the incentive to keep going was supplied by the teams. You can find out where your local club or group is by writing to me (with a stamped addressed envelope) at 6 Aldridge Road Villas, London W11 1BP, marking the envelope 'Clubs' or 'Aerobics', as appropriate to you.

## What is 'aerobic' exercise?

In answer to the first question, there is almost no such thing as an intrinsically aerobic or anaerobic sport or activity. It all depends on how the game is played and on the condition of the player. Because it is too leisurely, cricket is about the only outdoor sport involving activity that is bound to be anaerobic. (For fast bowlers it is anaerobic because the activity is too brief.) Of course, bowls, snooker, darts and similar recreations are not aerobic.

Other sports, such as football, hockey, basketball and squash, are aerobic only if played rather eccentrically, in continuous movement. Men who bring their competitive urges to the squash court and flail around, imagining that sweat and exhaustion are proof against the excesses of their everyday lives, are making a mistake. Squash played that way is anaerobic and will develop speed and strength but not endurance. Also, played fast, it is safe only for the highly fit person; played sporadically by someone with a sedentary job, it is fairly dangerous. Tennis and badminton are, by their nature and if played with some skill, more likely to be aerobic.

By their nature judo, boxing, karate and yoga are unlikely to be aerobic. Circuit training and downhill ski-ing can only be aerobic for the exceptionally fit person who can keep going without stopping for ten minutes. Weight training can be aerobic only if carried out on special equipment such as Nautilus machines.

If you are a recreational skier you may imagine that you can regularly ski for ten minutes or more without a break. Next time you are on the slopes, time yourself.

The recreations most likely to be aerobic are brisk walking, preferably in hilly country, and dancing. 'Aerobics' is also sometimes called 'aerobic dancing' simply because it is a form of dancing specifically planned to be vigorous for continuous sessions of about ten minutes. Golf can be an aerobic exercise for older people, not when playing a shot but while walking between shots. If a golf cart is used the sport cannot be aerobic. Carry your clubs!

The best aerobic exercise is any exercise that can conveniently be sustained for ten minutes or more at a time. In Great Britain jogging is the 'best' aerobic exercise simply because it is cheap, convenient and possible any day of the year. (For the beginner, a combination of walking and jogging will be aerobic; for a more experienced person, running.) Swimming is better all-round exercise, because it uses the whole body. The disadvantages of swimming are practical: access to pools, crowds, chlorine, the difficulty of swimming for ten minutes or more without a break. Cross-country ski-ing is the best aerobic exercise of all, and champion cross-country skiers have the highest aerobic capacity of all sportsmen and women. If this book were being written for a Scandinavian audience I would recommend cross-country ski-ing as the best whole-body aerobic exercise of all. Elsewhere, the problem is access to snow on flattish country.

An out-of-condition sedentary person, perhaps overweight, middle-aged and with a history of breathlessness, may well find any sport or formal exercise too hard at first; brisk walking may be quite taxing. Someone in this condition would certainly be out of breath walking up flights of stairs. If this describes you, be patient! Go for walks of ten minutes and more at your own pace, and don't think of taking more vigorous exercise until you feel ready. As the members of *Fun Runner '82* discovered, the body is remarkably resilient and develops quite quickly in response to exercise.

The second question I am most often asked is: 'How can I discover when my heart rate is elevated to 60 to 80 per cent of maximum?' Dr Cooper's estimate of 150 beats a minute applies to younger people, because maximum heart rate is a function of age. Roughly speaking, maximum rate is 220 beats a minute minus your age. For example, at the time of writing I am 42 years old, so my maximum rate is 178 beats a minute: that is about as fast as my heart will go. Thus younger people have faster maximum rates than older people.

The way to find out whether you are exercising aerobically is to take your pulse, at the wrist or if you prefer at the neck, with a watch with a second hand, immediately after exercise.

This drill is a feature of every well-organised aerobics class. Remember that the exercise should take five minutes at the very minimum: increase it to ten minutes or more as soon as you can. It is best to take your pulse for ten seconds the moment you stop exercising and then multiply by six. Heart rates for people of different ages are as follows:

| Age | maximum rate (minute) | 60 to 80% rate (minute) | 60 to 80% rate (10 seconds) |
|---|---|---|---|
| under 25 | 200 | 120–160 | 20–27 |
| 26–30 | 195 | 117–156 | 20–26 |
| 31–35 | 190 | 114–152 | 19–25 |
| 36–40 | 185 | 111–148 | 19–25 |
| 41–45 | 180 | 108–144 | 18–24 |
| 46–50 | 175 | 105–140 | 18–23 |
| 51–55 | 170 | 102–136 | 17–23 |
| 56–60 | 165 | 99–132 | 17–22 |
| 61–65 | 160 | 96–128 | 16–21 |
| 66 and over | 155 | 93–124 | 16–21 |

There are two other ways of determining whether exercise is aerobic. Since neither involve a watch or taking the pulse, however, they are less precise. The 'perceived effort' test (also called the 'Borg scale' because it was developed by Gunnar Borg at the University of Stockholm) requires practice and some self-knowledge. The effort required of exercise is rated on the following scale, from 6 to 20:

6
7  very, very light
8
9  very light
10
11  fairly light
12
13  somewhat hard
14
15  hard
16
17  very hard
18
19  very, very hard
20

Aerobic exercise should feel 'somewhat hard' or 'hard', corresponding to 12 to 16 on the scale. This subjective judgement can be verified by checking to see that it relates to a heart rate of 120 to 160 beats a minute. With practice, it is easy to judge without a watch that light or very hard exercise is anaerobic.

The third way of checking whether exercise is aerobic is the 'talk test', which is most useful during a jog. During aerobic exercise you should be able to have a conversation, albeit somewhat staccato, with a companion. If you cannot talk during exercise then it cannot be aerobic and will be ineffective, your heart rate is likely to have soared well above 150 beats a minute and you will be in 'oxygen debt'. The result will be that you will have to slow down to an aerobic level of exercise, or stop.

Unfit people often worry unnecessarily about the possible dangers of exercise. The body has ways of foiling people who try too hard. Exhaustion is its first defence. Anybody who persists in exercising too hard is then likely to get injured or depressed. 'Jogger's Blues' is a well-known condition that results from following a training programme designed for an athlete, not an ordinary citizen. Injuries should always be seen as a helpful warning sign. Do not continue to exercise if the pain of an injury gets worse or if the pain is sharp. In such cases see a sympathetic doctor.

To some extent aerobic exercise can be built into a healthy life. Walk to work or to the station; walk up stairs; cycle to work. Some of the women who graduated from the *London 1982/50* and *Fun Runner '82* projects now run to work and have insisted on the installation of showers.

### How much exercise?

The third and fourth questions I am most often asked are: 'How long should I exercise, each day and each week?' And: 'How long will it take for the exercise to have a good effect on my health?'

Strictly speaking, the answer to the fourth question is: it depends. The exercise programmes for which I have been responsible—*London 1982/50*, *Fun Runner '82* and, later, the *Sunday Times Getting in Shape* project—have lasted between five months and a year. The most remarkable changes in the completed projects happened about three months after the training began. Men and women of different ages found that their shapes changed (as measured by estimates of body fat, a better gauge than body weight); that they slept better and often needed less sleep; that they enjoyed eating and drinking what they liked; that they gained a natural sense of well-being (and were less inclined to continue with a course of drugs or psychoanalysis); and that they were recovering an enjoyment of their bodies and of playing and striving with other people that they assumed they had lost at the end of childhood.

I asked some participants to tell me what had happened. Michael Innes, a relatively fit 28-year-old:

> Running represents a personal challenge. Eight weeks on from the first tentative steps there has been no great metamorphosis; just a feeling of well-being and a remedy, perhaps, for mental fatigue after a day's work.

Terry Bennett, a 41-year-old solicitor who lost a couple of stone observed:

> I love those magic mornings when a mile into the run you feel good, and you know this is a day when you can push yourself almost to your limit for mile after mile, and you finish physically tired but mentally exhilarated.

He was writing about runs in winter, before breakfast and a day's work. Peter Bird, a 57-year-old insurance underwriter and a veteran of several marathons, had been a diabetic who some years before had decided to save his own life by running. He wrote, of a time when he was 4 stone heavier:

> I used to roll off the train at Charing Cross in the morning feeling dizzy with high blood pressure. I honestly believe that if I hadn't been encouraged to run, seven years ago, I would be dead by now.

Liz Parry, a 29-year-old teacher training, not for a marathon, but for the *Fun Run*, wrote:

> I am frankly amazed that I am improving in ways that I thought were personally impossible.

Vivienne Coady, a young mother of two children, found liberation:

> Once we have put in a couple of miles, I feel really great. I never feel tired; rather, a feeling of being refreshed. When I have felt tired before the run, I no longer feel so, afterwards.

She became a trainer for the *Sunday Times Getting in Shape* project as a way of giving to others what she had got herself. Don Clark, a 41-year-old probation officer, ran for another reason, to raise £10,000 for another machine like the one that had saved his life: a long operation had disentangled a cyst from his spinal column. He ran not to save his own life, but those of others. He found that:

> Running is peaceful, and it represents a kind of freedom. It establishes warm bonds between people. Part of me fell in love with the hippy ideal in the 1960s. The best parts of running allow me to relive the best parts of that.

The reply I enjoyed most came from James Kelly, a 49-year-old local government officer from Swansea:

> I felt lethargic and content to let life pass me by. Then in 1978 I joined in the first Sunday Times National Fun Run. Suddenly I was no longer one of life's spectators. Even the youngest typist was no longer looking at me as if I were her father. Success at last!

People who diet want to stop. People who persevere with an aerobic exercise programme do not want to stop.

The answer to the third question is that the Royal College of Physicians recommend twenty minutes of exercise, three times a week. Dr Cooper and Professor Wood have found that lasting health benefits occur at a rather higher level: they both recommend 80 to 120 minutes of exercise a week, preferably in four sessions. For a jogger this is the equivalent of a total of a gentle 8 to 12 miles a week, covered perhaps on two days during the week and the two weekend days, the sessions being as evenly spaced as possible. At this level profound changes in the cardio-respiratory system start and continue.

The US Health and Social Services Secretary Richard Schweiker said in 1981:

> By taking five simple steps, by not smoking, by using alcohol in moderation, by eating a proper diet and getting the proper amount of

exercise and sleep, a 45-year-old man can expect to live 10 or 11 years longer than a person who does not make these choices.

The hundreds of people of all ages I have run with, talked to, and corresponded with in the last three years have taught me that the first step of these five is exercise. The others follow as a result of exercise. And 'proper diet' turns out to have nothing whatever to do with dieting: for most people who exercise regularly, a proper diet is eating as much good food as they want to eat.

### More oxygen; more food

Why is aerobic exercise so special? First of all, because it is aerobic exercise that speeds up the body and increases our metabolic rate. Doctors and scientists who have not found that exercise produces this effect have not studied aerobic exercise.

Oxygen is the fuel for our internal fire that burns food. The more oxygen that is supplied to a flame, the brighter and faster the flame burns; this is as much true within the human body as it is within a grate. The action of a bellows enflames a fire; the action of the lungs, themselves a form of bellows, sends oxygen into the bloodstream for use in the conversion of food into energy.

The greater a person's capacity for oxygen, the higher the metabolic rate of that person will be. The more oxygen that is supplied, the more food the body can burn. To be more precise, there is a relationship between the oxygen intake of a person and the volume of food they require, in order to be in energy balance. The more fuel, the bigger the fire.

Food and oxygen combine to make the human fire. Most studies of energy balance look at food, or at oxygen, but not both. This makes only limited sense; the body cannot use one to sustain life without the other. The reason that the metabolic rate of the person on a diet or a fast goes down is not a mystery. The body balances a reduced food intake by reducing oxygen intake, and reduces oxygen intake still more when energy has to be taken not from food but from the body itself. Dieters train their bodies to require less oxygen. The main effect of diet regimes is to condition the body to tolerate diet regimes, which it does by a process of adaptation, lowering its metabolic rate, which is to say its use of oxygen. The more frequent and the more stringent the diet regime, the more dramatic and less reversible these effects will be.

It also follows that the body will balance a greater intake of food by taking in more oxygen, up to the point at which it has no more capacity. A very big man who is also phenomenally physically active will therefore have a gigantic appetite, but when as a result of change of habits or age or infirmity he ceases to exercise, much of the food he eats will turn to fat. This is because less exercise means less oxygen taken in, and less oxygen taken in means that energy balance can be sustained only if less food is eaten. Hence the dramatic fattening of Henry VIII and Edward VII when they stopped hunting.

The analogy with a fire in a grate is fair. Suitably ventilated, a small amount of coal burns bright and low; a large amount of coal burns bright and high. If a bellows is applied to a small amount of coal, more will soon be needed. If, on the other hand, little air can get to either a small or a large amount of coal, it will burn low, or not be burned at all.

Scientific studies of under-nutrition and over-nutrition are the key to understanding what dieting does to the human body. The body's use of the fuel, oxygen, varies as a function of the body's use of the fuel, food. As well as food, the body itself contains another fuel: fat. Just as food is burned with oxygen, fat is burned with oxygen. Dieting lowers the body's capacity for oxygen. Dieting therefore lowers the body's capacity to burn its own fat.

Since the ability to utilise fat as a fuel depends on the oxygen transporting capacity, the choice of fuel for the working muscle depends on the workload in relation to the individual's maximal oxygen uptake. The greater the maximal oxygen uptake, the greater the percentage contribution of fat to the energy metabolism at a given workload. Since training increases the maximal oxygen uptake, it also increases the facility for utilising fat as a source of muscular energy.

Which is to say dieting, by lowering the body's oxygen capacity, reduces the means whereby the body can burn fat as fuel. The passage above is from a classic book, *Textbook of Work Physiology*, by the Swedish physiologists Per-Olof Åstrand and Kaare Rodahl. Its implications are only now being assimilated into the study of obesity. The study of energy balance is the study not only of balance between energy taken in as food and energy used, but also of the balance between energy taken in from food and energy taken in from oxygen. In the energy equation, oxygen is not a 'given', a constant; it is a variable.

When energy from food outbalances energy from oxygen, fat is stored, and obesity is the result. Dieting reduces energy from oxygen and so is self-defeating. Over-eating increases energy from oxygen, which is, however, outbalanced by the extra energy taken in from food. The way out of this circle is to take in more energy without taking in more food: to apply the bellows of the lungs to the body's fire.

### The muscle that uses fat as fuel

Sustained aerobic exercise results in loss of fat and gain of lean tissue. In time its 'training effect' increases the metabolic activity of the muscles at all times. Another reason why aerobic rather than anaerobic exercise has this effect is that the two types of exercise affect muscles differently. There are two types of muscle fibre: red muscle fibre (also known as 'slow-twitch' muscle), used for work requiring endurance; and white muscle fibre (also known as 'fast-twitch' muscle), used for work requiring immediate reaction. Aerobic exercise uses red muscle, anaerobic exercise white muscle.

It is not known to what extent, if at all, exercise can alter the proportions of red and white muscle. But it is known that unused red muscle, that of a sedentary person for instance, degenerates into white-type muscle.

The fuel white muscle fibre uses is glycogen, the immediate source of energy stored in the muscle itself and in the liver. This store is essential and is replaced at the first possible opportunity, together with the water bound up with it. It follows that any weight lost through anaerobic exercise, which uses white muscle, will be from this essential glycogen and water, not from fat. This is why it is physically impossible to lose fat, or indeed to lose weight except temporarily, if you play squash, say, by thrashing around the court anaerobically.

Red muscle also uses glycogen. But, to take the analogy of a domestic fire, it does so not as its main fuel but as kindling. The chief fuel red muscle uses is free fatty acid, that is, fat released from the body's fat stores in liquid form into the bloodstream. Fat from the body's store is there to be used as fuel and of course, unlike glycogen, need not be replaced.

It is aerobic exercise—endurance work—that uses red muscle, and hence fat, as fuel. This is common sense. Aerobic exercise corresponds to the necessary work done by people who do not live in industrialised societies, such as Eskimos and Bushmen; or remote peoples such as Lapps; or peasants in the West, such as the country people of the Swiss Alps. These people do not gain weight or fat throughout their lives; they work aerobically at regular intervals; and they eat well. Even the most athletic hunter does not very often do the equivalent of playing squash. It is constant walking that wears away a stone or two.

Since unused red muscle degenerates into white-type muscle, the interesting if depressing consequence is that sedentary people gradually lose the wherewithal to lose fat. Thus the metabolic rate of the fattening person not only slows down, fat being less metabolically active than lean tissue; but the sedentary fat person also has less and less red muscle with which to use fat as fuel. This is undoubtedly the reason why doctors specialising in obesity do not usually believe in the value of exercise; and why the three very overweight women on the *Fun Runner '82* project got fitter but did not lose weight.

Fat sedentary people are liable to gain fat while eating moderately; and, having little red muscle, they have little chance to burn off fat by exercise.

The hard-hearted moral, and a warning to sedentary people who are now overweight and liable to become obese, is: don't get into such a state, or, if you do, learn to love it. But there is reason to believe that even obese people can convert white muscle into red by means of a course of gentle pre-training exercise. Such pre-training is unlikely to result in the loss of much weight or fat, but by regenerating red muscle it will give an obese person the means, with patience, with which to lose fat by aerobic exercise. In 1983 the *Sunday Times Getting in Shape* project is investigating this optimistic possibility with physiologist Malcolm Emery.

### A strong heart, a lively body

The effects of aerobic exercise on the function of the heart, lungs and blood vessels are well known. With sustained aerobic exercise, say for sessions totalling 80 to 120 minutes a week, the blood vessels enlarge and become more elastic. The heart, itself a muscle, becomes stronger and larger. Blood pressure drops. A further consequence is that resting heart rate drops, from say, the 'average' 72 beats a minute, to 60 and then down even further, to maybe 50.

Trained athletes often have a heart rate in the 40s. The average heart rate of the *London 1982/50* participants dropped to the 50s after marathon training. The simplest test of a healthy heart is resting heart rate; and it is very satisfying, knowing this, to find that heart rate drops, steadily, during a course of aerobic training.

At the same time, the heart also pumps more blood. Dr Kenneth Cooper estimates that an aerobically trained person will have up to two extra pints of blood in their body. This is because of a process of 'vascularisation' whereby blood vessels not only enlarge but also grow in number. The blood vessels on the surface of the heart itself may become larger and more elastic, and are therefore far less likely to be the site of a heart attack. Thomas Bassler, an American doctor, once claimed that running marathons gave anyone without a pre-existing heart condition 100 per cent protection against a fatal heart attack caused by irreversible blockage within a blood vessel. This claim is disputed, but there is no doubt that a runner's cardiovascular system is stronger than that of a non-runner.

It is healthier as well as stronger. Professor Wood, supported by other studies, has shown that high proportions of the abrasive, useful HDL lipoprotein are associated with aerobic exercise equivalent to jogging 8 to 12 miles a week. Below that level, exercise does not have a great effect on blood lipid levels. In California anyone can buy a customised car registration number: Professor Wood's is HIGH HDL, to remind people in the car behind of the good effects of running. Cholesterol is not in itself a health hazard. It is the type of fat in the blood that determines whether or not someone is at risk, and sedentary people tend to have high levels of the sticky LDL lipoprotein in their blood.

Aerobic exercise also promotes the growth of blood vessels close to the surface of the skin. This accounts for the healthy glow of runners and encourages rejuvenation of the skin. There is also evidence that aerobic exercise slows down or even reverses the tendency of bone to become decalcified and so brittle with age. Old people who break their bones as a result of a fall are usually sedentary people. According to the Royal College of Physicians:

> The need for middle aged and elderly people to continue to engage in regular and substantial periods of moderate activity each week runs counter to current practice. . . . There seems little doubt that the majority of adults in sedentary occupations are physiologically 'unfit' with poor cardiovascular responses to exercises.

New research is being done on the relationship of aerobic exercise and endorphin levels. Only recently identified and traced, endorphins are chemical substances whose structure is similar to morphine. Consequently they are sometimes known as 'the body's natural opiates'. There is some evidence that endorphin pathways are the pathways traced by acupuncturists, and so account for the otherwise mysterious anaesthetic effect of acupuncture.

Endorphins are released by the body under exercise—or induced stress—and may postpone the sensation of pain in physical crisis until the need for action has passed. They may be what enables a footballer with a broken collar-bone to score a goal, or a runner to complete a race with blisters.

There is evidence that smoking inhibits the flow of endorphins, replacing this natural process with the artificial soothing of nicotine; hence smoking's addictive qualities. There is also evidence that aerobic exercise 'jogs' the endorphins into action. So the way of stopping smoking may be to start aerobic exercise, not try to give up smoking, and see what happens. Half the *London 1982/50* and *Fun Runner '82* participants who started as smokers found that they stopped more or less spontaneously during the projects. They found themselves instead enjoying the 'jogger's high', the natural and intense sense of well-being of which endorphins are the source. Hence Terry Bennett's 'magic mornings'.

For people who are out of shape aerobic exercise is the way forward. Dieting will only depress an overweight person. We need more air. Aerobic exercise allows us to eat more while losing fat. In moderation, it puts the body in energy balance at a natural level, higher than that of a sedentary person, so that good food will provide enough nourishment. Aerobic exercise enlivens the alimentary tract and strengthens the cardiovascular system. It is the means to health through fitness.

### Table 3. Health Through Fitness

This aerobic training schedule is based on ten rules, seven stages, and 49 steps to be taken at your own pace, as it suits you. It will work for any able-bodied person whatever their initial state of fitness. Remember that it takes a long time for the body to get out of shape; so it will take some months to regain what you have lost.

### The Ten Rules

1. *Start at the beginning.* Whatever your initial state of fitness, start at stage 1. Do not move up a stage until you can complete every session in a week comfortably.

2. *Variety is the spice.* Some sessions are longer, moving from 10 to 40 minutes from stages 1–7; others are shorter, building up from 5–10 to 20–30 minutes.

3. *Rest as well as exercise.* Start with three and then four sessions a week, as shown, with rest days in between. (The chart assumes that weekend days are convenient; if not, of course other days will do as well.)

4. *One step and stage at a time.* Progress at your own pace. Don't force yourself to move from one stage to the next. The best test of your progress is a sense of well-being and energy after exercise.

5. *Backsliding is OK.* If you find a stage too hard, move back. If you get fed up or ill for a while, don't worry. Start a stage below where you left off. The same applies to holidays, but you will enjoy holidays more if you keep exercising.

6. *Train aerobically.* Walk-jogging, then jogging, is the most reliable aerobic exercise: it is simple , available, easy to measure. The two longer sessions should be jogging. For the other sessions please yourself with any aerobic exercise.

7. *Measure your own fitness.* At the very beginning, and every time you move up a stage, measure your fitness (by means of the system on page 186).

8. *First target is 80–120 minutes a week.* Stages 5–7 are where the cardiovascular benefits will take place, provided that your exercise is aerobic.

9. *Second target is 8–12 miles a week.* As soon as you reach stage 5, you are ready for the 'two-mile' test on p. 185. Use this to check that you are, when you jog, covering 8–12 miles a week or its equivalent in other aerobic exercise.

10. *Warm up and warm down.* Before and after every session stretch and bend your body, and jog on the spot or walk, for a few minutes.

There is no rule about how long it will take to reach stage 5: it all depends on you. If you treat the schedule as a competition and push yourself up stages you are fairly likely to injure yourself. As a rough guide, the majority of people I have worked with have taken 10–20 weeks to reach stage 5. If you reach stage 7 and want to go further, see 'Further Reading' on p. 242.

### The Seven Stages and The 49 Steps

|         | Sat | Sun | Mon | Tues | Wed | Thurs | Fri | Total |
|---------|-----|-----|-----|------|-----|-------|-----|-------|
| Stage 1 | **10** | — | — | **5** | — | 5 | — | 20 |
| Stage 2 | **15** | — | — | **5** | — | 10 | — | 30 |
| Stage 3 | **20** | — | — | **10** | — | 10 | — | 40 |
| Stage 4 | **25** | 10 | — | **10** | — | 15 | — | 60 |
| Stage 5 | **30** | 15 | — | **15** | — | 20 | — | 80 |
| Stage 6 | **35** | 15 | — | **25** | — | 25 | — | 100 |
| Stage 7 | **40** | 20 | — | **30** | — | 30 | — | 120 |

Days printed in bold are the days for jogging. All days left blank are rest days. The rest days are a vital part of the 49 steps. The figures are minutes. As long as the total for the week is right you can vary the length of any session up or down by a few minutes, but do not shorten the long run and do not cut out sessions.

*Measuring Your Own Fitness*

The sense of physical and mental well-being that grows, with aerobic exercise, is as good an indication of the development of health through fitness as any test a doctor can perform.

You will find it valuable and fascinating to measure the development of your health through fitness, by the tests overleaf. Carry them out every time you reach a new stage in the Seven-Stage plan.

The 'self-measurement' tests on the chart, you can carry out yourself. The way to measure your heart rate at rest and after exercise is explained on page 171. The 'fitness tests' are offered at some health clubs and doctors' clinics. Search them out; if you cannot find them write to me at 6 Aldridge Road Villas, London W11 1BP with a stamped addressed envelope marked 'Fitness Testing'. Have fitness tests done every three or six months if you can.

When you reach stage 5 find out how long it takes you to run two miles. Eight laps of an athletic track is near enough two miles; otherwise prepare a route on a large-scale map. Do the 'two-mile' test every month once you reach stage 5.

*Gear.* You will need shoes especially made for jogging. These have built-up heels and look a bit like landing craft. They are expensive. Do not skimp on them; they prevent injuries to the lower legs and knees. You will also need a tracksuit for cold days, and of course shorts and T-shirts.

## Self-measurement

| | Start | Stages: 1 | 2 | 3 | 4 | 5 | 6 | 7 |
|---|---|---|---|---|---|---|---|---|
| **Body** (inches) | | | | | | | | |
| Chest | —— | —— | —— | —— | —— | —— | —— | —— |
| Waist | —— | —— | —— | —— | —— | —— | —— | —— |
| Hips | —— | —— | —— | —— | —— | —— | —— | —— |
| Thighs | —— | —— | —— | —— | —— | —— | —— | —— |
| Weight (pounds) | —— | —— | —— | —— | —— | —— | —— | —— |
| | | | | | | | | |
| **Heart Rate** (per minute) | | | | | | | | |
| At rest | —— | —— | —— | —— | —— | —— | —— | —— |
| After exercise[1] | | —— | —— | —— | —— | —— | —— | —— |
| 3 minutes after | | —— | —— | —— | —— | —— | —— | —— |
| 10 minutes after | | —— | —— | —— | —— | —— | —— | —— |
| | | | | | | | | |
| **Two Mile Test** | | | | | | | | |
| Minutes/seconds taken | | | | | —— | —— | —— | |
| | | | | | | | | |
| **Fitness Tests** | | | | | | | | |
| Blood Pressure | —— | —— | —— | —— | —— | —— | —— | —— |
| Body Fat Percentage | —— | —— | —— | —— | —— | —— | —— | —— |
| Oxygen Capacity[2] | —— | —— | —— | —— | —— | —— | —— | —— |
| Fitness Rating[3] | —— | —— | —— | —— | —— | —— | —— | —— |

[1] immediately afterwards
[2] $VO_2$Max (ml $O_2$ min kg)
[3] Cooper scales

CHAPTER SIX

# The Woman Dieter

In this era, when inflation has assumed alarming proportions and
the threat of nuclear war has become a serious danger, when
violent crime is on the increase and unemployment a persistent
social fact, 500 people are asked by the pollsters what they fear
most in the world and 190 answer that their greatest fear is
'getting fat'.
KIM CHERNIN
*The Obsession*

'I suppose you really do believe that your happiness is consequent
on your size? That an inch or two one way or the other would
make you truly loved? Equating prettiness with sexuality, and
sexuality with happiness? It is a very debased view of sexuality
you take, Phyllis. It would be excusable in a 16-year-old—if my
nose were a different shape, if my bosom were larger, if my
freckles were gone, then the whole world would be different. But
in a woman of your age it is vulgar.'
FAY WELDON
*The Fat Woman's Joke*

### Fat is seen as wrong

Fear of becoming fat and desire to lose weight obsess women in
the West. As the Duchess of Windsor said, 'A woman can never
be too rich, or too thin.' In our society being slim is associated
with glamour, success and beauty. Slimness is felt to be the ideal
to which all women should aspire. The image of the fat man

retains an attraction, as an embodiment of power (Winston Churchill) or of joviality (Falstaff). But the image of the fat woman, the 'earth mother', has been rejected, in a culture that has turned away from the virtues she represents.

It is harder for women to deviate from society's ideals. Fat women are penalised far more than fat men. Fat girls are less likely to gain college places than thin girls, they are less likely to be given help of any kind, they are more likely—even than the disabled—to be rejected socially. And they cannot find fashionable clothes that fit them.

Fat is seen as wrong at a very early age. In 1978 three researchers from the University of Cincinnati College of Medicine presented a group of pre-school children with two life-size rag dolls, identical except in one respect—and found that 91 per cent of the children preferred the thin doll to the fat doll. And they also found that, although the small number of overweight children in the group correctly identified themselves as looking like the fat doll, they all preferred the thin doll.

In the same study the children were presented with line drawings of children of their own age, varying according to weight, sex and age: for example, a fat white girl, a fat black girl, a thin white boy. The children were asked to pick out which drawings they 'especially liked' or 'disliked' and those they thought were 'weak', 'happy', and so on.

All the children preferred the thin children. The investigators wrote: 'There were three substantial trends: to see fat girls and thin boys as anti-social, to rate boys as more competent than girls, and to describe thin children as more competent than fat children.' In other words, their peers mark out fat girls as inept and unattractive long before they have a chance to prove their talents and sociability at school and later.

Fatness, like skin colour, is seen by young children as a social stigma.

When shown pictures of children they actually knew, the pre-schoolers showed a significant tendency to relate heaviness and the anti-social items, but only for black boys and girls.

In a study undertaken in 1963 the nutritionist Professor Jean Mayer found that:

> When obese subjects demonstrate attitudes similar to those resulting from ethnic and racial prejudice, it is not far-fetched to say that obese persons may form a minority group suffering from prejudice and discrimination.

Women's fear of becoming fat, and their perennial dieting, springs from sources deeper than taste or fashion. In our society only thin is good.

## A personal tale

I became a devotee of the cult of slenderness when I was nineteen, in my first year at university. I come from a European family whose eating habits are un-English; at school, a London mixed comprehensive, we brought our own sandwiches for lunch, or went out. I expected great things from university. What I got—among other things—was my first experience of institutional cooking and communal eating. It was a shock.

In the first term, we had to eat breakfast in college. I was appalled, fascinated too, by the cornflakes, greasy fried eggs, mounds of baked beans and floppy white bread. I did what was expected of me, and tucked in. And in a strange new world, for those first few weeks, food was comforting. I felt sick and stodgy quite a lot of the time, but I had been brought up to eat well; mealtimes in my family were a recognised source of pleasure.

In eight weeks I gained 10 pounds. I was horrified. For the first time in my life I felt gross.

I came to loathe the smell of stewed cabbage and gravy, and began to associate the grey lukewarm meals with the girls who ate them. I shrank from the image I saw of hundreds of pasty faces wolfing down fodder. My fear, I now recognise, was of being swallowed up by the mass, of losing my own identity.

Eating punctuated every occasion. The cakes, the chocolate,

the teas and biscuits, the late-night cocoa, the furtive and not-so-furtive Mars Bars and Kit-Kats, as essays were written or confidences swapped! We were lonely and unhappy girls, stuck out in remote and draughty buildings, eating as compensation, not for pleasure. I was disgusted and miserable. One day there was only one pair of trousers I could wear. I panicked. This was not, could not be me. I had—I decided with compulsive urgency—to reject this environment.

I needed an image, an identity, that worked for me and was as distinct from those around me as possible. And so I decided to get thin. Returning for the second term, I began my campaign. I still remember my first evening back. I announced that I 'didn't want' dinner and went to bed early with a mug of hot milk, feeling excited, empty and nervous. I had been brought up to eat properly; this was a whole new experience.

I became good at calorie counting. Soon I knew the energy content of scores of foods by heart. Fruit, yogurt, crispbread and endless cottage cheese; salads; picnics in friends' rooms: these became my eating routine. As often as not conversation revolved around food and slimming. I read slimming magazines. Proper sit-down meals made me nervous. Life was busy. I cycled everywhere, and I became addicted to the process of slimming. I swung from highs to lows; from feeling on top, beautiful, in control to troughs of feeling depressed, weak, defeated. I came to associate the lows with 'feeling fat', and forced myself back to ever fiercer self-denial.

After a few days' fasting I would go back to my mouse portions of cheese and crispbread, with 'rewards' of chocolate. When I did go out to dinner, the next day was a day of penance. I loved being skinny. It was the mark of my self-control and my 'headiness'. I wore tight jeans and a navy Guernsey for nearly all my four university years to emphasise my streamlined image. And I was encouraged by other girls' remarks. 'How thin you are!' they said. I heard envy and admiration.

I wasn't aware how thin I had become; I rarely weighed myself. When my jeans were tight, I felt fat; as long as I remained at size 10 I was happy. I'm 5 foot 7½; at that time I weighed 8 stone 8 pounds, sometimes as little as 8 stone 3. I suppose I approached the state of anorexia nervosa. But I did eat regularly, even if the quantities were tiny, and I did eat meals when avoiding them would have meant embarrassment or confrontation—at home, for instance. Nevertheless over a period of six years I became very attached to my own habits, always preferring a snack to a meal—which also meant taking cake or a biscuit, as well as fruit, rather than protein or something cooked. My unexpressed fear was that if I ate normal meals regularly I would lose control, be swamped by my body.

I realise now that I kept myself permanently under-nourished. Looking back, my high times were memorable. But they were peaks rising from valleys of depression, listlessness, body-weariness. I got cold very easily. My digestion was bad. I suffered from anxiety. I suppose I assumed that these malaises were the human condition, woman's condition, or my personal bad luck. It did not occur to me that dieting was making me ill.

Later on in London, no longer living alone, I could not avoid meals. Gradually and with some pain, I began to recognise my fear of food as a neurosis. My obsession with a super-slim profile began to fade, but it took a long time to stop panicking as I put on weight, to stop assuming that I would be judged and rejected in terms of my weight, to stop putting an image before the needs, health and fitness of my body.

And I began to see, too, the irony of the obsession that so many women have with their weight today. It is taken for granted that to be attractive women must be slim. How remarkable that, at a time when women have never been freer to express their opinions and exercise their rights, they are most bound to constrain the shape and weight of their bodies, by dieting.

## Fear of fatness

The 1983 Royal College of Physicians' report on obesity cites a recent estimate that, at any one time, 65 per cent of British women are trying to lose weight; and that of the 31 per cent of the population who are regular users of one or more slimming products most are women.

Statistics indicate the extent of dieting. They cannot convey the emotional involvement or the cost in terms of money, time, energy and pain. The 1982 report of the *Economist Intelligence Unit* on health products states that slimming is no longer to be seen as a special activity separate from normal eating. We have moved, the EIU report judges, 'towards the concept of weight management as part of regular personal health care'. But for women, dieting is less a question of 'weight management' or 'health care', more a way of life.

Clair Chapman is an actress with the Spare Tyre Theatre Company, a British comedy cabaret group whose acts comment on the state of women and their bodies. Interviewed in December 1981 she said: 'I was put on a diet by my mother when I was 12. Dieting was an initiation into womanhood. I thought women just had periods and dieted.'

Many women have come to know the cycle of dieting and relapse, pounds lost and pounds regained, as intimately as they know their menstrual cycle. The discomfort of self-denial is followed by the guilt of eating again, and the body gradually becomes more and more flabby, not just in the mind, but in reality.

Katina Noble, another actress with Spare Tyre, said:

> I remember how humiliated I was when my boyfriend said I must get some weight off before we went on a holiday abroad. How desperate I felt, on going to a hypnotist and finding a money-grabbing charlatan. After eight years of this I was just so neurotic. I went up and down between 8½ and 12 stone, but I was just as suicidal at 9 stone 4 as I was at 11 stone 12. I went to such lengths to cover up! Making sure the upper arms weren't showing, never showing my bottom, not wearing trousers for six or seven years; I used to wear a skirt down to my ankles and a patchwork dress over it. My whole life was piles of clothes.

A turning-point precipitates many women into the dieting cycle. Very often this turning-point is adolescence, fear of the sudden curves, thighs and breasts of womanhood. Sometimes the crisis is pregnancy when their body not only contains another being but also gains weight fast. Post-natal depression compounds the alienation a mother may feel from her own body, and she may throw herself into a diet which fights her needs and those of her baby at just the time when, if she is breast-feeding, she most needs proper and nourishing food.

Other women diet because of approaching middle age. They refuse to accept that youth is past and focus on being slim as a way of showing that they remain attractive. For these women ageing is to be feared, in a society that prefers the freshness of youth to the wisdom of years. So often in middle age women become less active, subject themselves to chronic under-nutrition and lose their self-esteem.

Why do we see only slim women as beautiful? Why are anorexia nervosa and other eating disorders increasing? Why has dieting mania gone so far that the top 'non-fiction' best-sellers are diet books, in the USA and now in Great Britain as well? Why are women so uncomfortable with food and their bodies? Why, when dieters know or at least sense that diets do not work in the long term, do women continue to diet?

Traditionally, women have been denied the power to shape and control their lives. But they have enjoyed sovereignty in two areas: food and nurture, and beauty and the body.

Food, feeding, feasting, eating, cultivation, harvest: these are all concepts rich in meaning and ritual. Notwithstanding our mechanised world of fast food chains, baked beans and packet mash, everything that food stands for retains its symbolic meaning much more than we may care to realise. To offer food is still a primary act of hospitality, acceptance and love. And the principal responsibility for feeding, as for all other forms of nurture, has always fallen to women. The first food of life comes naturally from the mother's own body.

It is the woman who shops, cooks, feeds her man and her children. It is her responsibility to make food wholesome and appetising. Every day she provides for her family. Yet our culture teaches her to beware of feeding herself. Next to recipes for mouth-watering meals, magazines print the latest diet instructions. In one feature women are taught to create a miracle of meringue and cream; in the next to avoid the temptation of puddings.

What happens to a woman brought up on this double-think? Many become adepts. Others become what are now termed 'compulsive eaters': they eat neurotically, either too much or too little, in response to signals that have little to do with real hunger or appetite. These women become out of touch with their real needs and desires; their sense of control over the process of feeding themselves becomes shaky and intermittent.

Women who restrict themselves to 1000 to 1500 calories a day subject themselves to voluntary semi-starvation. The diet ended, the woman (and a male dieter too) is liable to fall on food with an intense and insatiable hunger that persists for a remarkably long time. This is why the dieter, ending the prison-like sentence of the regime, so often celebrates with what may very well be the first of another series of binges. But even if the dieter does not over-eat, in due course the old weight is regained.

Thus are the seeds sown for compulsive over-eating: uncontrolled eating of entire gateaux, quarts of ice-cream, shelves-full of food from the refrigerator, by night as well as by day. The dieter is aware of what is happening, finds no way to stop, and is full of despair.

### The new religion

These cycles of denial and reward, starvation and gorging, are familiar to many seasoned dieters. In *Fat is a Feminist Issue* Susie Orbach says that American women spend $10 billion a year on weight control methods. There are five chains of slimming clubs in Great Britain, all thriving, and more in the USA. In the United Kingdom Weightwatchers alone runs 1400 classes every week. In the USA the Diet Workshop runs 14,000 groups where 45,000 people meet weekly. Late in 1982 *People* magazine reported on the Cambridge Diet, a soluble powder sold at mass rallies by 177,000 'counsellors' throughout the USA who make $6 on every $20 can.

One after another they rose to testify. 'We are part of a fresh spring rain to wash clean the body of mankind' enthused one of the faithful. 'He is Julius Caesar' wept a follower, referring to the leader. 'He is everything! Isn't he gorgeous! Our leaders do love us! This is a magnificent church!'

Dieting is taking on the forms of religion: churches, prophets, bishops, priests, confession, surrender, redemption, and communion celebrated not with bread and wine, the symbols of an age-old meal, but with chemicals. Slimming clubs report that 90 per cent of their clientele are women. The readership of slimming magazines is similar. *Slimming*, once published and edited by Audrey Eyton, author of *The F-Plan Diet*, and the most successful of the six British slimming magazines, has a circulation of 321,000.

Women's therapy centres have now been founded in London and New York. The Centre in London reports that a quarter of the calls it receives every week are about eating problems. One letter in *TV Times* provoked a mailbag of 800, all from women asking for help with eating problems. Almost 90 per cent of the patients of a special clinic solely for eating disorders set up in Cincinnati in 1977 are women, and all are extremely distressed by their apparent lack of control over eating behaviour. In some cases the eating patterns they exhibit are quite deviant from the normal population, but often they are unremarkable, except for the tremendous guilt they engender.

Woman's second domain is beauty and the body. And it has often been well said that the ideals of beauty set for women, and the fashion industry that every year makes new rules for the game, are both a function of man's impulse to limit woman's development. For beauty gives women power over men; indeed, seduction can be a woman's prime weapon. But the battle is lost before she begins, for beauty takes much maintaining, and beauty, alone of the instruments of power, wanes with age.

There is the twist: by adoring the physical beauty of women, men turn women into their own jailors.

Of the 1001 people whom *Which?* magazine interviewed for its *Guide to Slimming*, 58 per cent of the women wanted to slim for cosmetic reasons, only 19 per cent of the men. The women who were dieting for their looks were also the least overweight. Rather than concerning themselves with their health and fitness and with encouraging an inner beauty, women have—certainly until very recently—been preoccupied with gilding their cages. They spend vast sums of money on cosmetics and clothes, on polishing, manipulating, admiring and pummelling their bodies.

For both men and women, the female body, naked or clothed, is the most potent icon of our civilisation. In our sitting-rooms we become as familiar with the world depicted on television as we are with our own, real, world. By and large women on television are uniform. They are almost invariably of 'normal' weight and shape, and slender. The average soap opera or family show portrays women who are slim and polished and usually have a supportive role—as wife or mother or nurse. In leading roles women combine head with heart, but heart—or rather, as often as not, the 'needs' of a man and the home—wins out.

For adolescent girls the message is confusing. Be bright and independent but not too independent, for the 'real' woman is a man's woman. Be seductive, but let the man be dominant. Be slender, but keep the kitchen stove bubbling and the home fires burning. And if, throughout this juggling act, the woman remains immaculate, well-groomed, then success, fame and happiness can be hers.

In Great Britain alone, over ten million images of women naked to the waist are printed every day in popular newspapers. The female body is everywhere—on billboards and magazine covers, in shop window displays, selling rum, car radios, double glazing, cheese, insurance and rust remover. As we wait for a train our eyes are forced to wander over bits of women displayed on posters—Pretty Polly legs, a Lovable body, a Colgate smile, Silvikrin hair, the Lee bottom. The images and the fantasies that go with them say: use our product, look like this, and men will pay up. Be beautiful and be bought chocolates and jewels, be wined and dined, be bedded and married and happy. Like the products her body is used to sell, woman becomes a commodity on the market. She is both bait and catch.

A woman is aware that her own body does not compare well with the bodies on the posters, which encourage her, as they do men, to see female bodies as objects. Jo Spence, a photographer who collects images of women, has observed the fragmentation techniques used by advertising agencies. In Gina Newson's film *Body Images*, made in 1981, she said:

> You get on one page a pair of lips, you turn over and there's a pair of legs; turn over and there are eyes: turn over and there's a face that's been hacked in half by the edge of the page. It turns the woman into a fetish. She's completely ripped out of time. A little bit of her comes to represent her, in the image.

It is hard for women to see themselves whole. Neither, very often, do men see women whole. 'I'm a bum man.' 'I'm a tits man.' 'I go for legs.' Women also fix their attention, less cheerfully, on parts of their body. 'My bottom is too big.' 'My nose is all wrong and my bosom is too small.' 'My problem is my lumpy thighs.' Men and women think of women's bodies as a collection of parts. Living in an age when defective parts of machines, and now defective organs inside the human body, are pulled out, thrown away and replaced, women have a constant sense of inadequacy about the 'defective' parts of their body.

## The self-hatred syndrome

Many women come to hate their bodies, and try with the help of doctors to treat their 'defective parts' literally as if they were machinery. In 1979, 300,000 American women had their breasts enlarged, usually with silicone implants; and every year between 15,000 and 20,000 American women have their breasts reduced in operations that frequently fail and leave them grossly disfigured. Barbarous methods of losing weight have now been devised. By-pass surgery to remove a portion of the intestine is usually followed by severe, prolonged and repulsive gut problems and can kill. Stapling, an operation that closes off the upper portion of the stomach with sterilised staples, is also dangerous, and the staples are liable to tear.

Jaw-wiring has been in the news in Great Britain recently. This is a procedure which requires a woman to live on a liquid diet for a year or more, with her jaws wired shut. Any woman put on this regime will of course lose weight, and after a while she will learn how to talk, after a fashion. Cases followed up after the jaws have been unwired usually show massive and dramatic weight gain. The following report appeared in the *Sun* in January 1983:

> Hairdresser Lynne Oakley, who shed 10 stone in two years, has put most of it back on again—in two months. The wires doctors put on her jaws to stop her eating snapped before Christmas—and so did her willpower. Lynne, 30, who tips the scales at 24 stone, said yesterday: 'It happened at the worst time when everybody was eating and drinking'. She was down to 15 stone when she abandoned her battle of the bulge. Now she's going to start again.

The long-term 'success' rate of jaw-wiring is not known, because it is a new technique. Probably most women who subject themselves to jaw-wiring will in time regain the weight they lost.

Most of the women who submit themselves to these procedures are grossly obese, to the point at which their lives are in danger; or their obesity prevents some other surgical operation. But in the USA some by no means obese women have found doctors willing to carry out these procedures. What causes the self-hatred that drives women to these drastic ends? It is not merely because their bodies do not conform to current standards of attractiveness. Such women have come to think of their bodies as 'things'. A young girl in Gina Newson's film says:

> I remember hearing this poem once, by Leonard Cohen. He was writing about his mother. He said 'She viewed her whole body like a

scar grown over some earlier perfection'. And I knew what that meant as if I'd written it myself, I knew from my soul. There's some very nice 'me' inside and it's just spoiled by the way I look. I feel so fat and ugly.

The girl was shown in silhouette; she could not bear to be seen. Gina Newson told me that she was normal size, even on the slender side, and was in no way ugly.

For women fatness means ugliness, and to be ugly is to be rejected, lonely, on the margins of society. And so, by an appalling association of ideas, some girls and women who are lonely and feel rejected come to believe that this is because they are ugly and fat, even when by any sensible standard they are no such thing. No wonder women go on diets.

A woman is taught to think of her body as a thing separate from her inner self. And yet she is also taught that her body is her means of expression. Boys are brought up to direct their energies outwards; girls are trained to project their personalities by means of physical attractiveness.

In her book *Why Women Fail,* the psychiatrist Ann Dally writes about self-destruction. This, she says, is one of

the biggest handicaps that women face today. It reveals an inability to choose constructively in a world of choice or to find a positive way out of dilemmas created by choice. Even time-honoured female preoccupations such as catching a man are liable in our society to be self-destructive.

In dieting, women turn their energies in on themselves, often in fear and distress, and concentrate on the private safe world of their own body—but which then, when the diet fails, they feel has let them down too. Dieting begins as a comforting occupation which avoids conflict and engagement with the unknown, the world outside, and then becomes a new and inescapable ground on which battles are lost.

These wars start early. The young girl with anorexia nervosa uses her body both as an object of her own will and as her one means of self-expression. Abandoning interaction with her family and with the world, the anorexic girl holds tight to the only territory which she feels to be her own: her shrinking body. Some anorexics say they would rather die than give up this control. Some do die.

Although anorexia is defined as a disorder separate from dieting, many anorexics begin by dieting. And a severe diet undertaken by a girl whose normal food includes a lot of junk may induce pathological loss of appetite for biochemical reasons alone. However it may be triggered though, anorexia nervosa is not a disease but a neurosis, a severe maladaptation caused by circumstances which are common to all women. Cases of anorexia nervosa are increasing, and are no longer confined to adolescent girls from a middle-class background.

In her classic work *Eating Disorders: Obesity, Anorexia Nervosa and the Person Within*, Professor Hilde Bruch outlines hundreds of case histories. Anorexics, she says, tend to be above average in intelligence, and speak lucidly about their feelings. One girl whom Professor Bruch was treating said: 'This was something I could control. I know my body can take anything.' Another, by contrast, was afraid of being strong: 'Her ideal was to be weak, ethereal and thin, so that she could accept everybody's help without feeling guilty.' For Sheila MacLeod, who has written of her own experience in *The Art of Starvation*, being plump suggested being fattened for the kill; alternatively, being swallowed up by family, school and university.

For some women, becoming thin is a bid for autonomy. The woman with developed pathological anorexia goes so far as to deny anyone access to her when they offer food, or the comfort and love associated with food. This contrasts markedly with the dieter, who wants to fit in with society's standards. Anorexics lose any real perception of body size; in their diminishing world they cannot see that they are becoming skeletal.

New eating disorders are now being identified. The latest to hit the headlines of the women's pages is bulimia. Bulimics have a normal body weight which they maintain by vomiting, as often as two or three times a day. Some women settle on this means of controlling their weight and use it for years. So too do some sportsmen who must keep their weight down—jockeys, for example. Bulimia, which is painful unless you have developed stomach muscles, eventually strips teeth of their enamel and soaks the digestive system with acid. Vomiting to avoid weight gain is a practice that the bulimic will keep secret. It isolates her, in our society, even more than the taking of illegal drugs.

A single small announcement was placed in *Cosmopolitan* asking bulimic readers to complete a questionnaire. Over 1000 replies were received. Over half this number of women made themselves vomit at least daily; about 70 per cent were generally disturbed; 89 per cent had 'profoundly disturbed attitudes to food and eating'. Although most of the women felt they needed medical help, only 30 per cent had mentioned their habit to a doctor. Bulimia is not often noticed, because sufferers usually have a normal weight, and the need for secrecy, and the sense of shame and disgust they feel, keep them underground. Magazine articles in which women talk about having been anorexic are quite common nowadays. But I have yet to read a piece about a woman saying that she throws up and is proud of it.

## Women, food and society

There is something horrifyingly wrong with a society that drives women to diet constantly, to starve themselves beyond help, to void their food. These conditions are commonplace in our society.

The condition of women preoccupied with their weight is pitiable: they blame themselves, punish themselves; allow themselves to be subjected to 'aversion therapy' in which they receive an electric shock when confronted with chocolate; conditioned by slimming clubs to re-train all thoughts about food; told that their instincts to nourish and be nourished are bad.

Women are taught to be afraid of food. For dieters the fear develops because diets do not work and increase the desire for food. Many women are caught in a trap which makes food, the source of life, that which is most to be feared. No wonder that so many women have 'disordered' eating habits.

Priests and doctors have put the weight of their authority on the side of body-hatred. Within Christianity the spirit is at war with the flesh and, since the Fall, it has been woman's flesh that has tempted man into evil. The Virgin Mary, pure and beautiful and often depicted as slim, is not an exception and proves the rule—for, unlike any earthly mother, she is a virgin. In *The Second Sex* Simone de Beauvoir writes:

> The flesh that is for the Christian the hostile *other*, is woman. In her, the Christian finds incarnated the temptations of the world, the flesh and the devil. All the fathers of the church insist on the idea that she led Adam into sin.

Christianity associates woman with the earth, with the old pre-Christian religions and so with the devil, whom Christians pictured as a perversion of the horned gods worshipped before Christianity in Europe. Women who understood the ways of the earth, knew the plants and herbs that would restore well-being, heal wounds and help in illness were labelled witches and destroyed, and much of their knowledge with them.

In the Middle Ages and well beyond, Church and state both enforced fear and suspicion of woman's body. 'Get thee to a nunnery,' Hamlet says to Ophelia, who goes mad. Othello eventually believes that Desdemona is lustful and murders her. Chastity belts, female circumcision, convents, chaperones were all means used to protect men against the supposed carnal impulses of women, and to protect women against themselves.

Rampant suspicion of women's sexuality lay behind many so-called 'scientific' beliefs propounded by doctors in the nineteenth century. The *Journal of the American Medical Association* in 1894 recommended treating sexual desire at the menopause with hot douches of up to ten quarts daily and leeches to take fluid from the region of the uterus. The physician's conclusion sounds much like that of a modern diet doctor: 'Such patients have so much lack of confidence in themselves, their physicians and their friends, that they have not the willpower to keep up a systematic course of treatment.'

Writing in 1910, Havelock Ellis found that the belief, spread by doctors as scientific orthodoxy, that men and women breathed differently—men 'abdominally' and women 'thoracically'—stemmed from the fact that the women measured had crushed their stomachs with corsets. In *The Unfashionable Human Body*, social historian Bernard Rudofsky says: 'The physician, whose business it is to keep us in good working order, was then as reluctant to interfere with fashion's dictate as he is today.'

Jane Fonda to her cost found that Rudofsky was right when, as a model and then as a film star, she not only dieted obsessively but, to force her weight down, took drugs for over ten years.

No doctor ever told me of their side effects. No doctor ever took the time, or showed enough interest, to ask just how and why we were using these amphetamines. Nor did any doctor warn us that we could become addicted to them—as I did.

Today, food has replaced sex as the focus of women's disgust and guilt. It is fatness that leads to damnation: slimness through dieting is the salvation.

The dos and don'ts of the diet books are the new dogma, the lists of forbidden and allowed foods the new catechism; and the diet doctor replaces the priest and physician of the past as woman's guide to grace. When organised religion is absent other rituals take its place. It is no accident that dieting is most widespread and diet doctors most powerful in those countries, mostly Protestant, where religion has lost its grip. And, just as Christians are taught that their bodies are vessels of sin and that salvation is through faith, so dieters can come to believe that their struggles and their failures only prove the need constantly to discipline and punish the body.

The futility of dieting fuels some women's sense of worthlessness. Others diet because they feel that as long as they are fat—in their own eyes—their life has not started, and that dieting will solve their problems. 'When I am thin, then . . .'—I will be beautiful, or healthy, or lovable, or happy, or successful, or effective. The *Which? Guide to Slimming* gives sober counsel to its readers:

> Losing weight will not of itself guarantee that you will find a marriage partner or improve your relationship with the one you have. You should regard your slimming as a rational task which will result in weight loss—not as a magic solution to all your ills.

### The fragile ideal

Has woman's flesh always been despised? By no means. The image of the Earth Mother has its origins in agriculture. It was women, there is little doubt, who first tilled the soil, planted, sowed and cultivated the earth, and gathered in the harvest. When settled communities began to be established, it was the women with flesh who were best protected against times of famine, most healthy, and most likely to bear healthy children. Fertility symbols often take the form of depictions of grossly fat women.

The connection between beauty and the promise of fertility and fecundity has been made for centuries in art. The paintings of Rubens and Rembrandt, and later of Courbet and Renoir, all celebrate the abundance of female flesh and a voluptuous sexuality.

In Europe, slenderness in women was first desired in the eighteenth century. In the Age of Enlightenment, the emerging middle classes had less fear of disease, plague and famine were no longer rampant, and the food supply was more assured. Man required a companion on his now extended journey through life.

The woman of leisure came to be associated with the finer things of life: with art and literature, taste and refinement. Sense and sensibility were the hallmarks of an ideal marriage partner. The wife of the peasant continued to be buxom; the wife of the gentleman was sensitive, her elegantly slender body betraying little sign of the basic functions of life, her soft white hands giving no sign of work, her delicate complexion unmarked by weather. That, at any rate, was the image, the ideal, of female slenderness.

As the concept of companionship implies, women were being raised from an entirely subordinate role to one of greater equality, one more 'like men'. And, of course, the male physique—translated to a woman's body—is slim. In her book *Fat and Thin*, medical historian Anne Scott Beller says:

> People tend to ape their betters, and women's aspirations to the unmodulated physiques of men express unvoiced, and until recently probably largely unconscious, judgements about the nature of male status and privilege compared with their own.

The *grandes dames* of the Parisian *salons*, famous for their wit, charm and intelligence, had posed a certain threat to men. Thereafter, the second image of the ideal female shape did not so much develop out of the first as parody it.

The nineteenth-century lady was fragile and languorous, liable to fainting fits and to the vapours. Her vulnerability emphasised the strength, power and superiority of the man. The pallor of a Dame aux Camélias was a sign of an all-too delicate constitution. Consumption became chic. This ethereal creature did not so much diet as starve herself. She was too unworldly for such coarse matters as food. She took enemas and purgatives to maintain her tiny waist. Her tightly laced corsets made sure she could not digest food properly when she did eat. Her body weak and crushed, she often miscarried. That, at any rate, was the image to which so many Victorian women were expected to aspire, and their failure, as their bodies resisted their regimes, must have made them as guilty and ashamed as any female dieter today.

In *Illness as Metaphor* Susan Sontag says:

> Twentieth-century women's fashions (with their cult of thinness) are the last stronghold of the metaphors associated with the

romanticising of TB in the late eighteenth and early nineteenth centuries.

## Independence or vulnerability

Since the early 1960s—years in which the contraceptive Pill has removed the risk of pregnancy from sex, and the woman's movement has grown—dieting has engulfed the women of the West. In some respects the compulsion to diet is similar to the contrasting forces behind the ideals of slimness prevailing in the eighteenth and nineteenth centuries. Today, some women diet to assert their sexual freedom, seeing the sexually active body as lean, smooth and honed. Others, by contrast, diet to show an appealing vulnerability, seeing the submissive body as slim, soft and petted. These opposing ideals can resonate against each other, causing new confusions. An unpleasant recent example is the rise of the child model and movie star, the adolescent bodies of Brooke Shields and Jodie Foster becoming sex symbols in *Pretty Baby* and *Taxi Driver*.

Women's bodies, or rather the images of ideal women's bodies, are on show everywhere. Ever since Twiggy's astounding success as a model in Great Britain and the USA, millions of women have half starved themselves in futile attempts to achieve her figure.

Attractive women are seen as young and slim, and therefore many older women have found themselves neglected, rejected and abandoned by their husbands—traded in for a younger model. Many such women, preferring to lose their dignity rather than their man, have starved themselves into scrawny versions of their post-adolescent rivals. Hilde Bruch comments:

> It is impossible to assess the cost in serenity, relaxation and efficiency of this abnormal, overslim fashionable appearance. It produces serious psychological tensions to feel compelled to be thinner than one's natural make-up and style of living demand. I do not know how often people are aware of the emotional sacrifice of staying slim.

As time passes women very often find that, unless they exercise, the only way they can stay slim is to submit to a state of perpetual semi-starvation, perhaps also to take drugs, and are quite likely to form extremely disordered eating patterns. The consequence is depression, exhaustion and illness, and a reduced life expectancy. In these circumstances it is better to fail. Professor Bruch continues:

> There is a great deal of talk about the weakness and self indulgence of overweight people who eat 'too much'. Very little is said about the selfishness and self indulgence involved in a life which makes one's appearance the center of all values.

We all need a sense of control over ourselves and our lives. But we have lost a sense of control, restraint, mastery. Anything goes; the bomb may drop; redundancy is round the corner. The woman who chooses not to restrain her sexual appetite is likely to transfer her need for some form of restraint on to food. Other women diet just in order to be able to hold some sense of order. The language women dieters use to describe their fears is significant. 'I mustn't let myself go.' 'I'm afraid of my fat taking me over.' 'My body's out of control.' 'I feel helpless when I gain weight.' The rituals of the diet regimes, with their lists and numbers and orders of the day, are a sure sign of a general malaise. The sad irony is that dieting itself creates the alienation from the body, the weakness, illness and flabbiness that the dieter most fears. Dieting is now the most widespread self-destructive activity known to woman.

Mastery is a male concept. The women most concerned to prove themselves the equal of men, in men's domains such as business and industry, are particularly likely to see pencil thinness as the sign of dynamism, mind over matter, and a rigid armour typical of the male executive. The image is not that of an earthy siren—a Dorothy Lamour, Marilyn Monroe or Sophia Loren—but of heady adventuresses such as Bette Davis, Joan Crawford and Katharine Hepburn, mannish, independent and tough.

Other women try to make sense of the demands put on them, and the demand they put on themselves, to be both independent and also good wives, lovers and mothers, to work well in the office and at home, to satisfy colleagues, man and children. Such women too are liable to be driven into themselves and seek control by dieting, just as much as the adolescent.

Dieting is liable to be an attempt to compensate for the lack of control women feel over their lives. Women from all walks of life and all classes feel confused because of conflicting desires to be mother, home-maker and also independent people with their own lives, and are liable to retreat into the one area they think they can control: their bodies. Sadly, defeat in dieting is likely to be the most inevitable defeat of all.

The swings from self-denial to self-indulgence, from fasting to feasting—all of which may involve secret or furtive eating—reflect women's oscillation between her conflicting roles. For the younger woman the pressure is more than ever to be thin. The Superwoman image cultivated by Helen Gurley Brown of *Cosmopolitan* and by Shirley Conran in Great Britain is an image of both femininity and independence: these women represent themselves as having it all ways. 'If only I could look like that,' other women think, go on another diet, and fail again—and again.

Self-doubt, anxiety, lack of confidence, confusion, self-destructiveness: these are emotions most women know all too well. Successful women too: 'Will I be lovable if I'm strong and independent?' 'Will my children hate me for having a career?' 'If I choose to stay at home and care for my family will I regret it later?' Women's magazines are full of questions like these.

Many women turn to dieting as a ritual; as a pattern of behaviour designed to stop growth, to live within 'rigid boundaries', even as a way to stay within emotional adolescence.

Women are now becoming more free not only in their minds but in their bodies also—with much hesitation. The realisation is dawning that dieting is a lonely and frustrating business that usually fails; and also that the rules of the calorie charts, the instructions of the diet doctors, the obedience and submission involved in dieting, the fragility and weakness that come with loss of weight are all repulsive as well as futile.

As they turn away from spending their lives being told what to do, women should also turn away from the regulations and restrictions and, yes, the persecution of dieting regimes and diet doctors. Men are more and more discovering the value of their emotional selves. Women have the opportunity to discover the strength and power of their physical selves.

This does not mean opting for the Earth Mother image, which is just as limiting as the Slender Superwoman stereotype. But it is time to abandon the notion that a woman needs to be – should be – thin to be the best or proper kind of woman. It is time that this adolescent image is seen for what it is, and for women to find out what is the best shape and size for themselves as individuals. It is time, too, to abandon the costly and futile wars that women fight against their own bodies, to abandon the diet regimes that weaken them, depress them, and eventually—ironically—make them fat.

It is time for women to get on the move.

# CHAPTER SEVEN

# The Active Woman

It is vain to say human beings ought to be satisfied with tranquillity: they must have action, and they will make it if they cannot find it. Millions are condemned to a stiller fate than mine, and millions are in silent revolt against their lot. Women are supposed to be very calm generally; but women feel just as men feel; they need exercise for their faculties and a field for their efforts as much as their brothers do; they suffer from too rigid a constraint, too absolute a stagnation, precisely as men suffer.
CHARLOTTE BRONTË
*Jane Eyre*

What is now called the nature of women is an eminently artificial thing, the result of forced repressing in some directions, un-natural stimulation in others. It may be asserted without scruple, that no other class of dependents have had their character so entirely distorted from its natural proportions.
JOHN STUART MILL
*The Subjection of Women*

### Finding yourself

For women exercise is the surest way to self-discovery and self-realisation. Accustomed to see themselves, and be seen, as passive, many women find the effects of exercise a revelation. Interviewed in San Luis Obispo, California, for *Running* magazine, Alice Werbel spoke of her first running steps, age 57, and after her husband Ernie had retired:

Your children are gone; you must get up and do something. We started to take long walks. We walked by the High School track, and one day I said – why don't we run, just a quarter mile or so. Then one day, we got to run a mile.

That was in 1973. The first race Alice entered was the 10,000 metre run at the Senior Olympics held at Irvine. Her son had sent her a wool warm-up suit and, knowing no better, she ran the race under the Californian summer sun wearing it. Afterwards she was told that her time of 53 minutes was a world record for women aged between 55 and 60. In 1981 she held six world records, for distances between 800 metres and the 1-hour run. In 1983, at the age of 68, she said: 'I so often wish that people could understand that they had it within them. You feel sometimes that you shouldn't be out there training on the track; that you should be in a rocking chair.'

At 8 in the morning on Sunday 29 March 1981 Sue Goggin, a 40-year-old mother of three, was at the gates of Greenwich Park to watch the start of the first London marathon. 'Oh what admiration I had for all those people, especially the old. If they can do it, so can I at 40,' she wrote. She started to jog—finding at first that she couldn't run fast enough to catch the bus to work. Then she joined the *London 1982/50* group, training to complete the second London marathon, on Sunday 9 May 1982; which she did, in a time of 4 hours 57 minutes. For her, running has given her a new freedom: 'It is marvellous to shut the front door and leave all the hubbub and squabbles of three children behind—let Dad sort it out for a while, and feel the freedom of running with one's own thoughts.'

Helen Johnston, a woman of 28, was part of the same London marathon team; she finished in 4 hours 21 minutes. For her, changed shape, not weight, was a benefit of running:

My weight has stayed much the same, although I eat more. Running makes me so hungry! A lot of women complain about flabby thighs. Mine used to be, but running has firmed them up – also backside. I just feel so healthy and fit!

## Calm and zest

Helen also found just how much many men need to believe that
women are and should be passive creatures, objects of admiration
but not active, energetic and strong. She was the victim not only
of verbal sexual aggression from men as she passed by on the run
but also of threatened physical aggression.

> Most scary are the kerb crawlers. I have nightmares of being dragged
> into the car. Then there are the pedestrians. The men are the most
> threatening and the most crude. All this upsets me, makes me angry,
> and sometimes I have honestly been very frightened.

When she started to run, Helen did not know how to handle this
kind of bad experience. But once her body was in training she
answered back.

Women report various benefits from exercise: sleep becomes
deeper, period pains subside, they feel calmer and gain zest.
Lucilla Deane, another young member of the London marathon
team, said:

> Physically I just felt more alive. I've always been rather a bad sleeper
> and suddenly I find, now, that I go out like a light. I felt that my body
> was using its food more efficiently. I don't feel hungry for at least an
> hour or two after a run. What I do eat I feel is being metabolised
> more efficiently now.

Some psychologists in the USA are discovering the
effectiveness of exercise over conventional psychoanalytical
methods in raising personal awareness and dealing with anxiety
and depression. In her book *Women and Sports*, Janice Kaplan
describes the work of Dyveke Spino, once a clinical psychologist
and now an Olympic coach, who uses physical activity in her
work with groups of women. Referring to the Greek ideal of the
integration of mind, body and spirit she says: 'You can't deal
with the mind and emotions unless you pay attention to sports
and games.'

Using movement therapy and jogging and running, she

encourages women to get in touch with an energy they were unaware they had and to find an untapped inner strength and vitality: 'Most women have a lot of self-doubt and built-in masochism. They don't really know themselves, and don't know how to go into the world and grab what they want.'

A run can be just as effective a therapy for depression as a session on the couch. An American psychologist, interested in the benefits of jogging, gave one group of people conventional analysis for an hour, one by one; and took a second group out together for half an hour's run. The joggers showed more improvement in their general sense of well-being and control over their lives; and they saved a lot of money, too.

## To own one's body

I began to jog, and then run, almost a decade after I became a student. I didn't choose to because it is the only suitable form of exercise; it isn't. But it is simple and convenient. In Great Britain you can run almost anywhere almost any time, and it's cheap: all you need is a T-shirt, a pair of shorts, running shoes, and a tracksuit for warming up and for cold weather.

For me the sensation of moving swiftly through the air unhampered by the usual layers of clothing, handbags and high heels, was extraordinary. On my first runs, just of 10 and then 20 minutes, I felt the flush of warmth through my body as my sluggish circulation started to work hard; and, afterwards, heaving lungs, tingling skin, the glow of physical exertion and later, the beginnings of real hunger. All these sensations, I came to realise, with a pang, are those of childhood. A long time before, and I didn't know when, I had put them aside, along with tree-climbing and make-believe.

Mobility is crucial to the growth process of children; it is the key to their sense of themselves in the world. We cannot know much about our bodies unless we move them; and this is why children are constantly on the move, touching and exploring the space around them and their place within it. Neurologist Paul

Schilder's work has shown him that when children stop moving they stop learning. This has special significance for the overweight and the obese. Commenting on Schilder's work in her book *Eating Disorders*, Professor Hilde Bruch writes, 'The inactivity so characteristic of obese people thus appears to be related to their often disturbed body concept.'

She is suggesting that some people become obese in part because of inactivity and, moreover, that inactivity is sometimes pathological, springing from fear of the world and fear of learning. Obese people often report feelings of alienation from their bodies; and their supposed calm and contentment is more likely to be a sense of powerlessness and anxiety about being active. Some obese people, women in particular, need a lot of encouragement to follow an exercise programme.

In the first months of running I made several other discoveries. My skin gained a bloom and glow. Quite soon I stopped puffing and gasping, as my body adapted to the new stresses I put on it. I felt that my lungs were expanding, learning a new rhythm of inhalation and exhalation which soothed me as I ran. Without becoming bulky my muscles started to become more defined and smoother, and my hair grew thicker and glossier.

I gained respect for my body, which I had so often distrusted and despised. I had no intention—nor have I now—of running races, let alone marathons; for me, running was and is for health and well-being. So as one running companion pushed me to run faster and longer, I moaned and complained: I was convinced that I couldn't do it, that I didn't want to do it, that it was too much for me. I resisted achievement with every technique. He was unimpressed; and to my surprise and—I must admit—pleasure, I found I could do it!

At school and university words were my means of expression; I avoided games at school, I am a poor and fearful swimmer and never learnt to play tennis. Sport was something sporty people did, so I was rather embarrassed to discover that I loved the experience and the effects of running. The world of physical expression is not one in which you can be smarter or cleverer; words don't come into it. It became a new way of being for me which I found exciting, liberating, and so a little dangerous and scary.

I began to test my new reliable body on runs of first two, then three, then four and a half miles. It no longer mattered that I thought my body was an odd shape; for I was enjoying it, being in my body rather than looking at it from the outside. For the first time since childhood, I had the sense that I owned my body.

Having run three or four times a week for a few months, I found a real and reliable sense of hunger. In the mornings I looked forward to my breakfast—muesli and yogurt and a pot of tea—but no longer needed to have lunch just because it was 'lunchtime'. I eat when I'm hungry. My appetite for starchy foods increased spontaneously, which at first worried me. But I now know that the active body needs a lot of unprocessed and unrefined carbohydrates. At the same time my appetite for meat, sweets, chocolate, alcohol and cigarettes decreased. I still eat cakes and have a drink from time to time, and the occasional cigarette; but I no longer treat myself to a pudding as a way of trying to calm some general sense of dissatisfaction.

I put on weight: about 6 pounds. The old part of me was horrified! But I was pleased with my body, and people kept telling me how slim I was: the catch-all compliment which often really means 'How well you look'. Loathe to part with old habits, I sometimes deprived myself of food, but then I came to acknowledge that the extra pounds belong to me, are part of my body as I feel it should be. And I recognised, and it was a shock, that what I used to label my neuroses—anxiety, depression, listlessness, hopelessness—were at least in part caused by years of malnourishment and under-nourishment. Angst is romantic, semi-starvation is not.

In any case, I was becoming pleased with the way I looked. My body composition changed as I lost some fat and gained some heavier lean tissue.

I started to enjoy listening to my body. For a while a series of malaises and infections made me feel as if running were in some way literally jogging poisons in my body to the surface. Whatever their cause, these illnesses ceased. Yoga classes, which

I had previously put off when I believed I had something 'better to do', became top priority; a couple of hours of stretching in a gym or an hour of running was never time wasted or lost, and gave me more energy and zest for my work. And I slept better.

The great surge of enthusiam for running, aerobic dance and many other forms of physical exercise among both women and men is not simply the result of a desire to get fit and to stave off heart attacks and middle-age spread. Exercise allows us to re-discover the child's joy of simply being alive. This priceless sense of well-being gives a sense of value to everything we do in life, and also a new sense of purpose. Running and dancing are a reaction against ways of life which any sensible person knows are too sedentary, too comfortable, too automated.

When I started to exercise in the open air it was not just the exhilaration of being energetic that spurred me on but also the forgotten joy of being part of the physical reality of nature. I had not realised just how much time I spent looking at the world through screens: windows; books, television, film; coats, hats and mufflers.

To run free with minimum clothing is a marvellous freedom. The world I got to know was that of Kensington Gardens and Hyde Park. I felt the different textures underfoot, tarmac, gravel, grass firm and muddy, snow. I watched the park grow as spring became summer, in different light and different weather. Wind and rain were simply that—cold and wet against the skin, bracing, not something to huddle up against. I felt the seasons change as shoots appeared, then leaves emerged emerald green, then darker in summer, then brown and gold in the autumn. I was within my own experience, as I passed by and came to know the people with their dogs, other runners whose route was clockwise, the tramp whose territory is a particular bench by the Royal Garden Hotel, the old lady forever painting the ornamental garden by Kensington Palace, from the east side of the vine arbour.

Exercising the body is a positive discipline, in contrast with the negative discipline of dieting. Any normal person on a diet longs for it to end. But once the body has become accustomed to exercise, a run, a dance session, a yoga class is something to look forward to: a freedom, not a restriction.

It all sounds simple and inviting. As Alice Werbel found, it is just a matter of being like a child again—getting up and running, or swimming, or dancing, for fun. But in practice for women there are more complex issues; Helen Johnston experienced one. And there are others: taboos, self-doubt, social demands, prejudice, inhibitions, prohibitions.

## Losing and winning

Women's attitudes towards sport influences their attitudes to exercise and physical activity. As they grow up, girls are encouraged to be more sedentary than boys. The very word 'tomboy' used, affectionately or not, of a girl nearing puberty speaks worlds.

Again and again girls and women are prevented from participating in sports regarded as men's domain. In Great Britain, the Equal Opportunities Commission championed the case of Theresa Bennett, whom the Football Association had prohibited from playing in an under-12 league. She won her case, but lost it on appeal. Evidence was put forward on Theresa's behalf that she was pre-pubertal and a 'guided missile in football boots'. Lord Denning set these pleas aside and refused further appeals, saying, 'We don't enquire about the age of ladies.'

Elizabeth Ferris, a doctor specialising in sports medicine, won the Bronze medal for diving in the Rome Olympics in 1960. At school her headmistress had her examined by a cardiologist on the grounds that so much training must be bad for a girl's heart. A less determined girl would have been discouraged. Kathrine Switzer is public relations director of Avon Products Inc. responsible for their involvement in women's running. In 1967 she entered the Boston Marathon, purportedly an 'open' event, as 'K Switzer', knowing that race officials would otherwise cancel her entry. In the event it took a hefty shoulder-charge from her boy-friend to prevent a race marshal manhandling her out of the race, which she completed.

And it was not so long ago that award-winning football writer Brian Glanville of the *Sunday Times* made it clear that in his view sport was all right for ladies but questionable for women: 'There is no reason why a woman should not indulge in any kind of sport she wishes.' (It's difficult to imagine a writer saying: 'There is no reason why a man should not indulge in any kind of sport he wishes.') Glanville goes on:

> A girl who goes out to run, swim, or play tennis for the joy of it is still being a girl. But a girl who slogs away all winter in a gymnasium lifting weights so she can beat other girls in the summer is behaving like an imitation man.

Winning is all right for boys. But a girl who wants to win—or even to exert herself to her utmost—is questioned. Rejecting a proposal that a woman's 3000-metre race should be included in the 1980 Games the International Olympic Committee said that it was 'a little too strenuous'.

No wonder that a recent survey in Great Britain showed that only 40 per cent of girls play any sports outside school and that half intend to give up all sport after leaving school. In contrast 70 per cent of boys played sport outside school and only 20 per cent intended to give up sport after school. The boys had been encouraged; the girls had been discouraged.

The image of the Olympic Games is the summit of athletic ability and the manifestation of the true spirit of sport, where to win is not so glorious as to take part. But Baron Pierre de Coubertin, founder of the modern Olympic movement, fought successfully to keep women out of the Games. Women's track and field events were organised separately from the Olympics in the early years of this century. A women's international meeting took place in Monte Carlo in 1921: over 100 women from five countries took part. The next year 300 competitors from seven countries participated, and it was decided to form a Women's World Olympics. After pressure from the 'Olympic Games' organisers the name was changed to the Women's World Games. These were held in 1922 in Paris. Men's track events such as the 400 and 1500 metres were reduced to 300 and 1000 metres. For the second Women's World Games in 1926, in Sweden, ten countries were represented in thirteen events. In his book *Catching Up the Men*, Ken Dyer observed that at this point women's athletics 'had grown from almost nothing to a major force on the sporting scene, with a programme almost as varied as men's and approaching theirs in level of participant support'. Only then was the perennial request that women be allowed to compete in the Olympic Games grudgingly accepted, for the 1928 Games. There were two conditions: women were only admitted provisionally and were confined to five events.

The all-male Olympic Committee thus effectively restricted what was becoming a flourishing and vigorous development. In the 1928 Games, held in Amsterdam, the 800-metre world record for women was broken by Lina Radke. As she and other competitors crossed the line, they collapsed from exhaustion. As a result the administrators banned all women's track races except the 100 metres, and thereafter the inclusion of every woman's track event had to be fought for. The 800-metre track event only reappeared in 1960, the year in which Elizabeth Ferris competed as a diver. Addressing a congress on women and sport in Rome 20 years later Dr Ferris said:

Even in 1960 only 600 of the 5,000 odd competitors were women, and they only competed in 6 of the 17 sports. We women, inside our very separate compound in the Olympic village, were savagely protected by patrolling guards who paced, panther-like, up and down outside a wire fence that was so high that not even the gold-medallist in the pole-vault could have got over it.

The women's 200-metre race was added in 1948, the 400 metres in 1964 and the 1500 metres in 1972.

The hardest struggle for women has been to gain acceptance for long-distance running events in the Olympics. It is only in 1984 that the 3000 metres and the marathon have been included. The absurdity of these delays is emphasised by the fact that it is in endurance events that womens' achievements are greatest. Ann Sayer recently took the all-comers' record for the 840-mile Lands End to John O'Groats walk, beating the previous record set by a man. (Asked how she managed to finish in thirteen days she said that she could only take two weeks off from work and had to be in the office the next day.) The American Penny Lee Dean holds the England to France cross-channel swimming record. Canadian Cynthia Nicholas holds the two-way cross-channel record. In 1980 Naomi James held the solo round-the-world sailing record. In long-distance, endurance events women have less upper body strength than men but compensate with comparable leg strength. And there is good evidence that in long-distance events women can regulate their body temperature better than men, and also that they use body fat as fuel more efficiently.

Avery Brundage, President of the International Olympics Committee from 1952 to 1972, was, in power and long service, to the Olympics movement what J Edgar Hoover was to American law enforcement. Brundage always made it clear that he, like any Victorian, was interested in ladies, not in women, in sport. He once said, 'I am fed up to the ears with women as track and field competitors. As swimmers and divers girls are beautiful and adroit as they are ineffective and unpleasing on the track.'

Discouraged at school, women are given inferior facilities at all levels. The 1981–82 allocation for the University of London Rowing Club was £7000. The club has a man's team and a woman's team, with equal numbers in each: £200 was allocated to the women's team. In all professional sports prizes for women professionals are far lower than those for men. But when they persevere and endure the training that makes champions, women are told they are 'unfeminine'. The great long-distance running coach Percy Cerutty had this to say: 'Who wants straight-legged, narrow-hipped, big-shouldered, powerful women, aggressive and ferocious in physique and attitude?' Clearly such a woman would be more than Percy could handle!

Common sense suggests that women have in certain respects powers of endurance superior to those of men: women's bodies are built to bear children. Miki Gorman was the first woman home in the Boston marathon twice, in 1974 and 1977, having her first baby at the age of 40 in between. 'Compared with having a baby, a marathon is easy,' she said. And during the 1970s, while the men's world record for the marathon remained at the 2.08.33 set by Derek Clayton, the women's world record was broken sixteen times, falling from 3.02.53 to 2.27.33. (In 1982 the records stood at Alberto Salazar's 2.08.13 and Allison Roe's 2.25.27.)

## Women are catching up

Why, then, is it only in the 1984 Games that the women's marathon has been accepted as an Olympic event? Elizabeth Ferris asked this question of a woman associate of the International Olympic Committee before the Moscow Games, at a time when thousands of women were competing in long-distance races. Eventually the reason given, said Dr Ferris, was that:

> She had seen a woman cross-country skier vomit at the end of a race, and this had offended her dreadfully. No woman, in her opinion, should be so exposed and vulnerable – it was against all her deeply embedded views about what it means to be a woman.

It is not only men's attitudes to women in sports that have held women back. Women, too, have resisted achievement. In Great Britain this attitude began to change dramatically in 1981. The staggering increase in interest in long-distance running triggered by the first London marathon in 1981 disguised an even more extraordinary commitment from women.

In 1978, according to statistics compiled by veteran runner John Walsh, just 1789 British people completed a marathon; of these, a mere 48 were women. In 1979 and 1980 Walsh kept records only of those who finished in a time of less than 4 hours; the ratio of women to men remained under 1 in 30. By contrast, of the 17,906 runners who registered for the 1982 London marathon, 1363 were women. Women are beginning to catch up; and women in Great Britain are catching up with a movement that started in the USA five years earlier.

The movement for fitness through sport is also becoming a movement for health through exercise. Early in 1982 co-author Geoffrey Cannon invited people with no previous experience of running to train for five months with the goal of completing the 20-mile *Sunday Times* National Fun Run. (This *Fun Runner '82* project is described in Chapter 5.) *Running* magazine, in which the invitation was carried, has a readership of at least four men to one woman. Yet more than half of the 130 replies were from women. One said: 'I desperately want to feel fit, healthy and mentally liberated from my two very adorable but demanding children. I would also very much welcome a challenge of this kind. Please be my saviour!' Another replied, simply: 'My ambition is to become fit and healthy.'

After three months of jogging, 38 Fun Runners were asked if regular exercise had affected their mood: were they more, or less, anxious or depressed, from time to time? This question affected the women very much more than the men. Of the 38, 21 said that regular exercise had definitely improved their state of mind. How much difference? This is how they replied:

| Bad mood, anxiety, depression | April | July |
|---|---|---|
| Every day | – | – |
| Most days | 8 | – |
| Most weeks | 5 | 3 |
| Occasionally | 8 | 10 |
| Hardly ever/Never | – | 8 |

I doubt that psychoanalysis would have such an effect so soon. And in July one Fun Runner decided that she would stop seeing the psychiatrist who had been treating her for some time—simply because she felt fine.

The well-being that comes from running and from other aerobic exercise takes different forms. The good effects of fresh whole food and of exercise are so simple, and yet so often they are profound. To my mind, the reason above all others for the astonishing rise in the numbers of women who now are physically active is not just the desire to get fit, stave off heart attacks or middle-age spread, or cure depression—although these are reasons, and good ones. The desire for action is the desire to rediscover the simple joy of being fully alive. The upsurge of running and dance is an appropriate reaction to our otherwise automated and sedentary lives.

'Energy is the power that drives every human being. It is not lost by exercise but maintained by it,' said Germaine Greer in *The Female Eunuch*. Ten years later Jane Fonda put Germaine Greer's thoughts into action, and the feelings of a new generation of women into words, in her *Workout Book*, saying:

> I do not claim that a strong, healthy woman is automatically going to be a progressive, decent sort of person. Obviously other factors are involved in that. But I am sure that one's innate intelligence and instinct for good can be enhanced through fitness.

Watching others transform their lives through exercise, women sometimes say, or think: it must be too late for me. The slinky goddesses on television putting aerobics classes through their paces can be a discouraging sight. But even at the highest levels of achievement women are discovering that age is not a barrier to performance. Joyce Smith holds the British women's marathon record and was seen on television by millions, finishing ahead of the other women runners in the London marathon in 1981 and again in 1982—when she was 44 years old. Beryl Burton, the long-distance cycling champion, continued to challenge male rivals well into her 40s. Mary Peters won the Olympic Pentathlon in Munich when she was 33. Miki Gorman continues to set world and American records for her age in the marathon. And for an older generation, the example of Alice Werbel, who started to jog when she was 57, can be an inspiration.

The time when her children grow up and leave home can be the time of a woman's life when she can use her experience and resourcefulness to discover a new taste for adventure, with an energy and steadfastness that many a young woman may envy.

It sounds simple. In some respects it is. Any able-bodied woman can get up and go running, or swimming, or dancing. But in ways that don't directly affect men, the progress of women is dogged by taboos, self-doubt, and inhibitions. It's not only the women athletes who have a hard time.

### Exercise and 'being a woman'

We adapt to the roles expected of us very early in life. Little children playing at mummies and daddies will act out the mother at home, washing-up, cooking, looking after the family; the father at the office being important, playing football with his mates at the weekend. Many television advertisements are versions of this game. No manufacturer ever sold a packet of soapflakes by showing the man of the house exclaiming with wonder at the whiteness of his wife's shorts as he fishes them out of the washer. Men are meant to be strong and independent; women are meant to be gentle and dependent: we are all taught that. A woman playing serious strenuous sport is as threatening as is a top woman executive; both women and men view such a woman as a challenge to the conventions of manliness and womanliness by which we live and limit our lives.

The sheer achievement of women tennis players, and their professionals' successful fight for prizes in line with men's has in some respects freed tennis from the pressures that discourage and inhibit women in other sports. Girls can look up to Chris Lloyd and Martina Navratilova as supreme athletes, fiercely competitive, and now possessed of some of the glamour once reserved for ballet stars.

In tennis and in other sports, though, the media give more attention to the good-looking woman who is not in the top flight. Stories are printed and rumours circulate about affairs, including homosexual affairs, involving women players, but not men; and it's all right for men players to be temperamental, short of John McEnroe, but the most protest women are allowed is a squawk.

A top male player is seen as attractive and admirable, and outrageous characters such as Jimmy Connors and Ilie Nastase are portrayed as lovable. But a top woman player—she's seen as a little bit strange; she is regarded with awe but also with some suspicion. She makes men, and other women, feel uncomfortable.

From time to time newspapers publish a story about a jogger who died of a heart attack, or, as a variation, about the jogger who was struck by lightning. Joggers have indeed been struck by lightning, but very rarely, and someone with a heart condition can, but also rarely, bring on a heart attack while running, although violent exercise such as squash is much more risky for someone with an undiagnosed heart condition. Readers still want to be told that jogging is bad for you; so the stories about people who die of heart attacks while sprinting for the bus, or in the midst of an unusually passionate embrace, go unreported.

Similarly, from time to time newspapers publish a story that women runners are liable to suffer from amenorrhoea (that is to say, their periods stop). Horror! The implication is that the woman loses her fundamental womanliness because of her sport. The message of this story is like the often told accounts of those tall high-jumpers and bulky hurdlers, usually from behind the Iron Curtain, who when tested turn out by some criteria to be male, not female! On the one hand, becoming athletic is liable to render a woman neuter; on the other hand, some women athletes are men anyway.

Amenorrhoea is a common condition, as often as not caused by stress. It is perfectly true that a woman who trains very hard, running more than 50 to 60 miles a week say, may find that her periods stop or become irregular, particularly if she is thin. The condition may be reversed by taking vitamin C and iron tablets, which are in any case advisable if she eats any amount of junk food and refined sugar. But there is no evidence whatever that amenorrhoea induced by very heavy training continues after the training is eased off. Why should it? Any woman runner who regards periods as a curse can see exercise-induced amenorrhoea as a blessing. Characteristically, though, the suggestion behind the newspaper stories is: don't jog, or you may not be able to have babies—a nonsense. Exercise does not turn women into men, and it does not turn women neuter.

After starting to jog, I spent time worrying that I would develop bulging muscles—just like a man. Again, it is true that some female field athletes and body-builders develop musculature like that of men, but only if they take anabolic steroids, illegal drugs that contain male growth hormones. Without drugs, not even women weight-lifters develop bulging muscles. I had allowed myself to be inhibited by a myth; I did not do what was obvious—look at the women athletes to be seen any week on television.

It is also true that exercise sheds fat and adds lean tissue, including muscle, to a woman's body. In action, the body of a woman who takes regular exercise is clearly toned; the shape of her muscle is unobtrusive, but it shows. Here a change in what is meant by beauty in a woman is taking place—and needs to take place. Exercise creates strength, and many men other than Percy Cerutty are made to feel nervous by women who gain physical strength. But, as women find just how good they feel about themselves after exercise, they discover an inner beauty which isn't painted on. Ken Dyer cites an interview with Anna Thornhill, an artist who is also a long-distance runner. She said:

> I don't worry about fitting in a fashion-type image any more. After running a marathon, and then a 7-mile race the next day and feeling no pains at all, I looked in the mirror and said, 'Body, you're okay. You're doing your job.'

And Ms Thornhill also referred to another issue that women face. What will my man think of the way I look?

> My husband doesn't want me to become too thin but I no longer want to surrender to someone else's view of sexuality; for me, functionalism and sexuality are fused. My sexuality isn't affected by the way I look any more, but by how I feel: healthy, confident and functional.

## The beauty of strength

Women, and men too, are finding out that a notion of beauty that depends on a softness which is a sign of weak and unhealthy fatness is not a notion of beauty worth holding; and that the firmness of the body and the inner glow that comes with exercise are more attractive and lasting.

Some women are put off exercise because they half-believe it will make them less of a woman. Others are afraid to exercise in public, either in a dance studio or in the open air, because they are only too well aware that they don't have the body beautiful of women in advertisements. Indeed, many women are afraid to show their body in private; sexual prudery often has little to do with morals, much more to do with fear of what the other person will think of the unclothed body. Privately, women often hug thoughts that they are ugly or clumsy, even deformed.

Having summoned up courage to join in a jogging group or an exercise class, one of a woman's first freedoms is to find that nobody looks like the women in the rum advertisements or the magazine fashion pictures. This is for the simple reason that these models, aside from having unusual shapes and exercising daily as most models now do, are also made up and lit and photographed from special angles, all to achieve an ideal effect which is not real. Stereotypes created by the camera, just as much as by the painter, do not exist in the flesh: meet a woman who is a model, and as likely as not her most attractive feature will be one regarded as a fault by fashion and so hidden in her pictures.

An exercise class gives a woman a chance to face her fantasies, including her own horrid fantasies about her own body, and realise that everybody looks different and that beauty is in the differences, not the similarities.

The second freedom for the woman who, at whatever age, starts to exercise regularly is that some of her features she dislikes and tries to disguise—dull complexion, flabby flesh, lumpy thighs—are liable to change, sometimes quite quickly, sometimes gradually. She begins to discover the natural shape of her body, a shape which, with exercise, she will begin to appreciate in new ways.

Physical exercise is not a panacea. It is hard work, and that is why the sense of well-being that comes from exercise is lasting: it is earned. People now are moving away from the idea of beauty that implies passivity, an idea that is a hangover from Victorian days. Slimness which depends on make-up, pills and diets has nothing to do with fitness or with health. As they enjoy the inner glow that comes from exercise, women today are contradicting the notion that beauty is only skin-deep. Diets treat the body as alien, as an enemy of the mind. Exercise treats the body as integral to us, as bound up with the mind and the spirit. After three months of jogging, Kathleen Herold, a 38-year-old member of the *Fun Runner '82* group, wrote:

> If I don't run every day my body lets me know that something is missing. I have lost weight, my blood pressure is down and my resting heart rate has lowered. Physically I am in better shape than I was 20 years ago; now I can run over two miles a day.

And Brenda Green, aged 52:

> If I'm driving the car and see a runner I'm tempted to stop and join in—and I'm so pleased to see more females running nowadays. I've now lost 10 pounds and big Sunday lunches are a thing of the past. I feel terrific: full of energy and confidence. I wish I had done all this years ago.

And the most engaging comment, in one of the newsletters the Fun Runners circulated to each other, came from Diana, the typist:

> I used to enjoy typing and I thought it was good exercise. At least I had fit fingers! But I have spent the last half hour typing about other people's running and thinking how much I would rather be out running than in typing. So I'm going to turn the typewriter off now and get my running shoes out!

At the end of the *Fun Runner '82* project Dr Barrie Gunter summarised the results: at the beginning and end of the five months, he asked all participants to complete a 'Cattell 16 Personality Factor Questionnaire'. The personality of the Fun Runners, men and women together, had changed significantly in five ways. Judged by the Cattell test they became more self-confident, more understanding of the needs and problems of others; less apprehensive; better mannered and less aggressive; and more relaxed and composed. Gunter was especially interested to note what had happened to the women:

> I believe that improved aerobic capacity can bring with it a feeling of well-being for the relatively unfit person—especially when he or she compares the way they feel now, with how they felt just a few weeks or months before.

Gunter emphasised that the most substantial shifts in personality occurred among women; for, according to his assessments, they started the project less self-assured, more tense and less emotionally stable than the men.

Given the pressure put on women right from the start of their lives to shrink away from their physical selves, these findings were hardly surprising. Wilhelm Reich has said: 'Every disturbance of the ability fully to experience one's own body damages self-confidence as well as the unity of the bodily feeling. At the same time it creates the need for compensation.'

At school, girls avoid each others' eyes, in the draughty changing-rooms, before and after the games they have to play. The scene is repeated later in life, in the changing-rooms of clothes shops. At school girls are taught that the 'sporty' girl, the female equivalent of the 'jock', is shallow and stupid. No wonder women so often start an exercise programme fearfully and look for excuses to fail or drop out.

What women are accustomed to is the world where chocolates and flowers and jewels are advertised as signs of love; where glossy magazines encourage fantasies of exotic places and exotic men; where less glossy magazines encourage daydreams of romantic passion. These treats are substitutes for joining in our own lives and creating our own drama, activity and excitement. Life is, should be, something we feel physically, experience through our bodies. And this is what women are now finding out for themselves. In October 1982 Pineapple Studios held a conference on 'The Exercise Boom' in London. Women of all ages from 18 to 70 came from all over Great Britain to take part. Aerobics, dance-exercise, popmobility: these are not fads confined to London and other cities. They are, all together, a new movement springing from and drawing encouragement from other and older disciplines.

### *A new harmony*

Thérèse Bertherat is a French body therapist who doubts the value of conventional forms of exercise that amount to drilling the body. She believes that an aerobic dance class run by a woman sounding like a shrill sergeant-major will only confirm a woman's fears that her body is inadequate. In her book *The Body Has Its Reasons*, Madame Bertherat writes:

> It is possible for you to find the keys to your body again, to find your proper vitality, health and autonomy. But how? Certainly not by regarding your body as a necessarily defective machine that encumbers you, as a machine made up of isolated parts, each of which must be entrusted to a specialist whose authority and verdict you blindly accept.

Yoga, too, encourages us to listen to what our bodies can tell us. So do other disciplines from the East, such as aikido and tai chi, and other forms of movement therapy developed in the West, including bioenergetics and the Alexander Technique. Some women will come to prefer vigorous, even exhausting exercise; the temperament of others will lead them into a quieter means to the same end. Barbara Dale, who runs the Body-workshop in London, teaches exercises which combine stretching used as 'active meditation' (in her words) with the aerobic exercise that the body needs to become healthy through fitness. She told me:

> I'm very aware that everything is reflected in your body. During the last 100 years we've come to realise that the mind is a tape of everything that's happened to you. People still don't realise that the body is the very same tape.

The aches and illnesses we suffer, the odd ways we have of sitting, standing, walking, are all part of our map, from which, if we are attentive, we can learn more about ourselves. As I kept on running, I also learned something that previously I would have dismissed as silly and perverse. I learned that discomfort and even pain can be valuable experiences which show what the body can bear; and I enjoyed exploring my limits, and finding that they expanded. Exercise that in one week would be uncomfortable, even painful, became easier in weeks to come, and so I wanted to try harder. How can we know who we are unless we know our limits? How can we learn about ourselves without exploring?

It is believed that the left hemisphere of the brain governs our reason and the right our intuition; and that we in the West have allowed ourselves to be dominated by the left half of our brain. All acts of creation require intuition to interplay with reason, and genius is always inspired by guesses that have nothing to do with logic. The free flow of energy that results from exercise seems to come from our intuitive, even psychic side, and the sense of well-being that invariably follows vigorous exercise may very well derive from a harmony between our two sides.

For women—and men—whose lives are packed with work, stress, decisions and conflict, exercise is the balancer, the healer. Barbara Dale also teaches relaxation, and she told me that:

> It's not super-fitness that keeps you healthy. That's fine to help you be more efficient but it's just as important to pay attention to relaxation: it's a very important part of fitness, health, and balance in every way. And if you're in good health you're much better able to cope with conflict.

People change and grow when it is required of them. Anyone who doubts the strength and resilience of women should recall what happened in both World Wars, when the women of Europe were needed as a new labour force. They took over heavy manual labour—welding, ship-building, machine assembly—previously done by men who before the war would have laughed at the idea of a woman doing 'their work'. It was not by chance that women's suffrage in Great Britain followed so soon after the First World War. As Vera Brittain says in her books, women who had worked in field hospitals in France were not prepared to be told that they were too weak and gentle to act as citizens. Even so, the progress of women's independence has been slow and faltering. After the Second World War public attitudes shifted once again when the men came back from fighting. Women were discouraged from working, with propaganda about 'eight-hour orphans'. Hair styles, fashionably short during the war and reflecting the fact that many women had practical work to do, became long, and as soon as dress material was plentiful Dior created the so-called 'New Look' which resurrected the wasp waist and cumbersome skirts.

The changes that are happening now in the USA and with increasing momentum in Europe have more general causes than war. Women nowadays are somewhat less inclined to listen to male voices of authority, whether these be fathers, bosses, priests, doctors or politicians. Women are more inclined than men to feel the futility and horror of a global arms system created by men. Some of the 30,000 women who in December 1982 encircled the Cruise missile base at Greenham Common, near London, said that politicians saw war as a game and nuclear bombs as their toys. The broad-based protest, especially strong among women, against the arms race and the threat of war is part of a general movement among women to make sure that their voices are heard.

Women are brought up to feed and care for others, to give their time, energy and love to supporting the activity of husband, children or boss. Many women feel uneasy, even guilty, at the idea of taking time to look after and nourish themselves. But just as no plant thrives without watering, no body flourishes without tender loving care, which is not always to be reserved for others. Women who take time each day to enjoy themselves in exercise, and also other forms of play, are less prone to self-destructive feelings of resentment and helplessness. People cannot fully love others unless they have self-esteem. Many women, busy with home and children, neglect themselves, not realising that a self-forgetful attitude breeds indifference and even contempt in others. No one ever thanked a wife or mother for saying, 'I did it all for you.' No wonder that so many women end up rejecting their tired, listless bodies, emphasising this dislike with the self-punishment, if not of drugs, then of dieting.

### Self-nourishment

It takes some courage for a woman to give herself time for self-nourishment. Any woman accustomed to dieting will at first resist the idea that good health and a reliable and lasting sense of well-being come from balance between our two fuels, food and air, and from plenty of both. It is hard to appreciate, at first, that the foods most often condemned by diet books—bread, potatoes, root vegetables, cereals and pastas—eaten in whole form are indeed the staff of life. New discoveries involve giving up old beliefs, and a woman who has spent 5 or 25 years dieting and in between diets will not find it easy to accept that her dieting was mis-spent time.

The self-nurturing and self-assertion involved in exercise go beyond good health. As they grow up girls are discouraged from being competitive and learn to disparage themselves, to compare themselves unfavourably with others. Many women deny that they are competitive because they have been taught to put themselves down, to feel that in any of life's races they will fail. Exercise encourages a sense of success; a woman does not have to come first in a sport to discover that she can achieve the physical goals she sets herself, then out-do herself. This self-realisation will dissolve the jealousies and frustrations that women so often come to believe are part of everyday life.

Another reason for changing health and well-being through good food and exercise is that women have found out for themselves that diets simply do not work. But millions of women, although they know that diets do not work for them, still believe that they are at fault, that they are weak, inadequate or greedy. This book is offered as a new freedom for all these women. Diets do not work: and it is their fault, not yours.

Through exercise women can become fit and confident, healthy and full of energy, and gain a new self-respect and control over themselves and their lives. And by learning to love themselves they will be able to love others better. By enjoying more of the good things of life, women can understand and discover themselves as whole people, strong, able, active, and in harmony with men.

# CHAPTER EIGHT

# *All You Need To Know*

It seems to me that we are still awfully ignorant of some basic biological knowledge regarding the nutritive value of food and its additives, its effect on the physiological activities of the gut, and the general metabolic consequences of this action.
SIR ERNST CHAIN
*Food Technology in the 1980s, Address to the Royal Society*

How we need that unity today, that glowing one-ness of body, mind and spirit! More than ever, now that the modern era of careless indolence and gluttony is so clearly ending, we need the tingling aliveness of every limb, the connectedness with nature and other people that only a full appreciation of embodiment can bring.
GEORGE LEONARD
*The Ultimate Athlete*

The thesis of this book can be summed up in thirty points. The first ten summarise the effect of dieting on the human body.

1   Diet books assume that the body works at a set speed; that some people have a fast metabolic rate, others a slow one, but that the basic rate for each individual remains the same. All the sums in diet books that tell dieters how many calories to consume are based on this assumption. It is wrong. Metabolic rate is not static; it is dynamic.

2   Diet books state or imply that most if not all weight lost on

a diet is fat. This is not true. The initial big weight loss advertised by many diet books as evidence of their effectiveness is of glycogen, a form of glucose stored in the liver and the muscles. Glycogen is the body's immediately available source of energy.

3   The weight lost on a prolonged diet is of lean tissue from the vital organs and muscles, as well as fat. The more severe the diet, the greater the proportion of lean tissue lost. Metabolic rate slows dramatically during a diet because much of the weight lost is of tissue which, unlike fat, is designed to be metabolically active.

4   The body of a person on a crash diet reacts as if to starvation; the body of a person on a prolonged diet reacts as if to famine. In each case the body will shed active tissue that consumes a lot of energy and as far as possible will protect the relatively inactive tissue making up the store vital at times of starvation or famine—fat.

5   The human body is more complex than that of any other creature and adapts throughout life to circumstances. The body of an active person will adapt to protect and develop muscle which is constantly used. The body of a sedentary person loses muscle as life goes on. The body of a sedentary dieter will tend to shed muscle because it is little used.

6   Glycogen is essential to the functioning of the body and the brain. Loss of glycogen triggers sensations of intense hunger, even if the stomach is full of food. When a diet is ended the body will replace its glycogen store. But the body of a sedentary dieter will tend not to replace all the metabolically active tissue that has been lost on the diet.

7   Constant dieting trains the body to endure diets. It does this by a process of shedding some lean tissue and replacing it with the fat needed at times of starvation and famine. Fat is itself

a source of energy and needs less fuel than the vital organs. The metabolic rate of the dieter tends to drop from one diet to the next, as the body adapts to need less and less food.

8 Loss of glycogen results in listlessness, depression and irritability. Loss of lean tissue, including muscle, results in the body needing less energy from oxygen in the air, as well as less energy from food, and coming into energy balance at a lower and lower level. Constant dieting makes a person feeble and torpid. This is a cumulative process.

9 A fat person may 'eat like a bird' and gain fat, because of a low metabolic rate caused by being fat. A lean person may 'eat like a horse' and stay lean, because of a high metabolic rate caused by being lean. Women need and use less energy than men; and a light yet fat middle-aged woman who diets regularly can gain weight even on a semi-starvation diet.

10 Dieting slows the body down and creates the conditions for gaining fat. Gradually, after one diet has ended, dieters get fatter and fatter on less and less food. Fat weighs less than lean tissue, and it is perfectly possible to lose weight as a result of accumulative diets and nonetheless gain a greater volume, as well as proportion, of fat to lean tissue.

This is why dieting makes you fat. The next ten points summarise why up to half the population of Western countries tends to get fat, with or without dieting.

11 Diet books imply that the basic requirement of the body is energy from food. This is wrong. The body adapts to very different levels of energy balance. The body's basic requirement from food is not for quantity but for quality. Above all, what the body needs is nourishment. What is wrong with the food we eat is not its quantity but its lack of quality.

12 Processed food lacks nourishment. During this century

people in the West have come to eat more processed, 'refined', sugar than any other food. Refined sugar is dead, or empty, energy. It supplies calories but no protein, fibre or vitamins and only a trace of minerals. 'Junk' foods supply energy but little or no nourishment. Refined sugar is the chief junk food.

13   Deficiency diseases are caused by a gross lack of nutrients. These diseases have mild forms that are difficult to diagnose, which may take the form of depression, exhaustion, swings of mood, anxiety, period pains, sleeplessness, irritability or irrational behaviour. One prime cause of such malaise, almost universal in the West, is eating junk food.

14   The body will always defend itself against the threat of illness. The body of a sedentary person who eats an average amount of processed foods and refined sugar will continue to signal hunger until enough nourishing food has been eaten. The only way for such a person to get enough nourishment from food is to consume too much energy from food.

15   Sedentary people gain weight and fat as a means of staying healthy. Overweight is not normally a cause of illness. But obesity (not itself a disease) is a cause of the 'Western' diseases, of the alimentary tract (including the stomach and digestive system) and of the cardiovascular system (the heart, lungs and blood vessels).

16   Some people eat much more processed food and refined sugar than others. People liable to suffer from deficiency states, or the 'junk food syndrome', for this reason include young office workers and housewives, students, people living alone, heavy drinkers, anyone with a 'sweet tooth', and anyone who eats only small amounts of fresh food.

17   Dieters are liable to be in a state of acute malnutrition as a result of the diet, unless they take great care to eat only nourishing food, including food rich in starch and fibre. Most

diets specify cutting out such foods, and it is almost impossible to avoid eating refined sugar, which is present in almost every type of manufactured food. Dieting can be a cause of illness.

18  After a diet regime has ended the body will signal acute hunger, as a means of replacing the nutrients of which it has been starved. This is the reason for the raging appetite and compulsive eating many dieters experience and is another reason why the body frustrates the dieter and becomes fatter after the diet. In the West, well-being often depends on being fat.

19  Refined sugar is worse than useless. As well as replacing nutritious food, it drains the body of some vitamins and is directly or indirectly implicated in various Western diseases. Eating refined sugar has the paradoxical effect of lowering the level of sugar in the blood. Sugar is a direct cause of diabetes, and is addictive. Eating sugar makes you hungry.

20  The body will always seek a level of energy balance at which the amount of nourishing food eaten will be sufficient for its needs. The body of anyone eating relatively small amounts of good food will therefore tend to slow down. Because people in the West eat a lot of food heavy in energy but poor in nourishment, they get heavier and fatter while eating less.

This is why people in the West tend to get fat. The next ten points summarise the means whereby we can lose fat and gain health.

21  A fire may burn bright with a small amount of good fuel and a gentle draught. With a strong draught a fire will burn faster and higher and use much fuel. As with a domestic fire, so with the human body. Human energy balance is between energy from food and energy from oxygen in the air. The more oxygen we breathe, the more food we will burn.

22  Dieting slows the body down, lowering the metabolic rate

as the body adjusts to need less food. Exercise of the right type speeds the body up, raising the metabolic rate as the body adjusts to need more oxygen and therefore also more food. The right type of exercise, using more oxygen, is 'aerobic' exercise, sustained at a point just below breathlessness.

23   Aerobic exercise creates a sense of well-being which is the opposite of the junk food syndrome. This is because anyone who exercises regularly will be eating more food and therefore more nourishing food. The body of the aerobically fit person will also develop a hunger for the nourishing foods it needs; whole foods, rich in protein, starch, fibre, vitamins and minerals.

24   Western life has deprived us of the regular exercise and also of the nourishing food that was enjoyed by people who lived well before industrialisation and that is now enjoyed by settled communities who live away from Western influence. As a rule such people do not get fat and do not suffer from Western diseases. We have much to learn from them.

25   A couple of hours of aerobic exercise a week, divided between four sessions, approximates to the work that peasants do as part of their lives. This exercise develops the muscle that uses fat as fuel and also strengthens the cardiovascular system. The result is a loss of fat, a gain of lean tissue, and a greatly reduced risk of various diseases, including heart disease.

26   Grains (including wheat, corn, rice, oats), legumes (peas and beans) and tubers (especially potatoes) are the staple foods of non-Western societies, as they were in the West before industrialisation. These foods are rich in starch, needed by the body and brain for energy, and also rich in protein, fibre, vitamins and minerals.

27   The importance of fibre, contained within whole foods, is that in effect it exercises the alimentary tract. In all respects food rich in fibre has the opposite effect from refined sugar on the

body. Eating whole food of the type that peasants eat is a vital part of an active life, and will lead to a greatly reduced risk of diseases of the alimentary tract.

28 Women have been taught to admire an ideal of slenderness, and to believe that dieting is the means to this end. Because dieting is self-defeating it reinforces the sense of defeat women often feel in a world run to suit men, and is damaging to women's mental as well as physical health. Women will gain self-respect by eating good food.

29 Women have also been taught to reject the ideal of strength, energy and competition, as being men's possessions. So women cling to dieting and resist exercise. It is time now for women to gain the freedom of enjoying their own bodies, to resist unreal stereotypes, and to gain energy, fitness and health by means of exercise that promotes a natural beauty.

30 Sedentary people in the West who eat bad food get fat and go on diets that do not work. Dieting is a Western perversion caused by bad habits that themselves lead to disease. The body is nourished by good food and regenerated by exercise. These are the principal sources of good health. We become fit and healthy by using all our energies.

# Further Reading

Here is a list of books and writers for the reader who wants to gain more information.

A recent account of overweight and obesity in Britain, recommending foods rich in protein, starch, fibre, vitamins and minerals, and also regular vigorous exercise, is:
Royal College of Physicians of London, *Obesity, Journal of the RCP*, January 1983

This follows an earlier American report of the McGovern Committee:
United States Senate, Select Committee on Nutrition and Human Needs, *Eating in America: Dietary Goals for the United States*, MIT Press, London, 1977

The group of British doctors who established the connection between processed carbohydrate (sugar in particular) and disease, and between unprocessed carbohydrate (rich in protein starch, fibre and other nutrients) and health, include Sir Robert McCarrison, Surgeon-Captain J L Cleave, Dr Hugh Trowell, Dr Denis Burkitt, Dr A R P Walker, Dr Kenneth Heaton and Dr Neil Painter. They are supported by Sir Douglas Black, Sir Francis Avery Jones and Sir Richard Doll. Anything written by these doctors is recommended, in particular:
Denis Burkitt, *Don't Forget Fibre in Your Diet*, Martin Dunitz, London, 1979

Denis Burkitt and Hugh Trowell, *Refined Carbohydrate Food and Disease: Some Implications of Dietary Fibre*, Academic Press, London, 1975

J L Cleave, George Campbell and Neil Painter, *Diabetes, Coronary Thrombosis and the Saccharine Disease*, John Wright & Sons, Bristol, 1969

J L Cleave, *The Saccharine Disease*, John Wright & Sons, Bristol, 1974

Sir Robert McCarrison, *Nutrition and Health*, The McCarrison Society, London, 1982

Royal College of Physicians of London, *Medical Aspects of Dietary Fibre*, Pitman Medical, London 1980

Four textbooks on nutrition, the analysis of food, and on vitamins and minerals, are:

A A Paul and D A T Southgate, *McCance and Widdowson's The Composition of Foods,* HMSO, London, 1978

The Staff of *Prevention* magazine, *The Complete Book of Vitamins*, Rodale Press, Aylesbury, 1978

The Staff of *Prevention* magazine, *The Complete Book of Minerals For Health*, Rodale Press, Aylesbury, 1981

Eleanor Noss Whitney and Eva May Nunnelley Hamilton, *Understanding Nutrition*, West Publishing Co., 1981

As this book goes to press, the *Sunday Times Getting in Shape* project, which I devised, is looking into the relationship between fitness and health under the direction of David Denison, Professor of Physiology at the National Heart and Chest Hospital in London. This is a new area of study, and there is no good up-to-date book on the subject originally published in Great Britain. Meanwhile, Dr George Mann, Dr Ralph Paffenbarger and Professor Peter Wood (in the USA) and Professor John Durnin and Professor Jeremy Morris (in Great Britain) have, with colleagues, published many contributions to scientific journals that are recommended.

The handbooks of Dr Kenneth Cooper, the pioneer of aerobic

exercise, are still valuable and include his own training programmes. These are:

Kenneth Cooper, *The New Aerobics*, Bantam, London, 1970
Kenneth Cooper, *The Aerobics Way*, Corgi, London, 1978

The best book for warm-up exercises, and general advice for the jogger, is:

Bob Glover and Jack Shepherd, *The Runner's Handbook*, Penguin, London, 1982

The jogger who intends to become a long-distance runner and run marathons should ignore the 'expert' training schedules of 60 miles a week. This is far too much. With the readers of *Running* magazine I have devised a schedule for runners who want to keep their health, friends and sanity:

Geoffrey Cannon ('Fun Runner'), 'The 88+1 Training Schedule', *Running* magazine, London, January, March, April, 1983

For women who exercise the two outstanding books for theory, history and practice are:

Ken Dyer, *Catching Up The Men: Women and Sport*, Junction Books, London, 1982
Jane Fonda, *Jane Fonda's Workout Book*, Allen Lane, London, 1982

Two books on exercise physiology are:

Per-Olof Åstrand and Kaare Rodahl, *Textbook of Work Physiology*, McGraw Hill, Maidenhead, 1978
William McArdle, Frank Katch and Victor Katch, *Exercise Physiology: Energy, Nutrition and Human Performance*, Kimpton, London, 1981

If you want a set of all the references used in the preparation of this book, please write to me, Geoffrey Cannon, at 6 Aldridge Road Villas, London W11 1BP. Mark the envelope 'DMYF references' and enclose £1 for copying, postage and packing.

# Index